THE TURNING POINT

MICHAEL D. STEIN AND SANDRO GALEA

THE
TURNING POINT

Reflections on a Pandemic

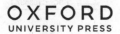

OXFORD
UNIVERSITY PRESS

OXFORD
UNIVERSITY PRESS

Oxford University Press is a department of the University of Oxford. It furthers the University's objective of excellence in research, scholarship, and education by publishing worldwide. Oxford is a registered trade mark of Oxford University Press in the UK and certain other countries.

Published in the United States of America by Oxford University Press
198 Madison Avenue, New York, NY 10016, United States of America.

Library of Congress Cataloging-in-Publication Data
Names: Stein, Michael D., 1962– editor. | Galea, Sandro, editor.
Title: The turning point : reflections on a pandemic /
Michael D. Stein and Sandro Galea.
Description: New York, NY : Oxford University Press, [2024] |
Includes bibliographical references.
Identifiers: LCCN 2023038581 (print) | LCCN 2023038582 (ebook) |
ISBN 9780197749685 (paperback) | ISBN 9780197749708 (epub) |
ISBN 9780197749715
Subjects: LCSH: COVID-19 Pandemic, 2020– |
COVID-19 (Disease)—Government policy.
Classification: LCC RA644.C67 T826 2024 (print) | LCC RA644.C67 (ebook) |
DDC 362.1962/4144—dc23/eng/20231012
LC record available at https://lccn.loc.gov/2023038581
LC ebook record available at https://lccn.loc.gov/2023038582

DOI: 10.1093/oso/9780197749685.001.0001

Printed by Marquis Book Printing, Canada

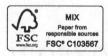

MDS: To Hester, Tobias, Alex, Roy, and Sofia.
SG: To Isabel Tess Galea, Oliver Luke Galea, and Dr. Margaret Kruk.

CONTENTS

SECTION 4. EMOTIONS

SECTION 5. THE FUTURE

PREFACE

During the COVID-19 years, we saw an intersection of multiple disruptions—a global pandemic, an economic collapse, and civil unrest that galvanized the United States and the world. Each of these alone would have been a shock to our collective system; together, they reflect an era that was truly unprecedented in recent memory. With the arrival of an effective COVID-19 vaccine, and widespread natural immunity, we managed to emerge from the traumas of those years. We are now able to reflect on the experience of a pandemic and ask ourselves how the lessons of that moment can inform a healthier present.

These lessons urge our engagement with the social, economic, environmental, and political forces around us. This means broadening our vision of health beyond a narrow focus on medical care. We need a wider understanding that a nation's policies and institutions are central to creating the conditions for health to flourish. These conditions include the quality of our neighborhoods, the state of our social safety net, and the health of our environment. Our failure to fully address these conditions led to our failure to mitigate the spread of COVID-19 to the degree we might have.

In *The Turning Point*'s essays, we look backward and forward. We ask: What lessons did we absorb during the pandemic that can guide us to the creation of a better, healthier world? In what ways did COVID-19 reveal mistakes that we are still making? What challenges did we see coming in the years prior to the pandemic but did not act on? What is the role of public health in creating a new status quo, one that integrates the lessons of the COVID-19 moment?

Throughout the book, we ground our engagement with these questions in lessons learned in real time during the COVID-19 years. We look at structural divides that appeared along the lines of race and economic inequality in 2020 and 2021. In doing so, we consider how they can be repaired or reconceived. We do so with the understanding that progress is never uninterrupted. Anything can happen at any time. When it does, we can hope it will be enough to motivate positive change. And we can do more than hope. We can have the conversations that help us learn the lessons of challenging times, so we can build a better, healthier future. This book is meant to help spark these conversations.

Michael D. Stein and Sandro Galea

March 2023

Boston, Massachusetts

ACKNOWLEDGMENTS

We thank Eric DelGizzo, Haradeen Dhillon, Meredith Brown, and Catherine Ettman, who made this book possible. We are indebted to the many members of the public health community who commented on earlier versions of the ideas presented in this book, helping us improve our thinking.

SECTION 1

LESSONS

THE COVID-19 moment provided ample lessons for how we engage with health in the United States and globally, pointing to the many ways our approach to health has fallen short. Creating a healthier future means learning the lessons of the pandemic and applying them to the work of creating a healthier world.

1

FROM THEORY TO PRACTICE

The long-awaited end of the COVID-19 pandemic was brought to us, largely, by vaccines. In a remarkable feat of 21st-century medical achievement, effective vaccines for COVID-19 were developed approximately nine months after the virus emerged, substantially faster than we had ever developed a vaccine before; the previous record for vaccine development was for mumps—and that took three years. Signals from vaccine makers—both those using the novel mRNA technology and those using more traditional adenovirus technology—had us anticipating the end of the COVID-19 pandemic as soon as the vaccines were available.

After a year that upended our entire economy, our collective incentives were aligned with vaccinating as many people as possible, as quickly as possible. Several professional organizations proposed guidelines for vaccine prioritization. The president set a target of 20 million people vaccinated by the end of 2020.

Then the vaccines arrived, and we faltered. By the beginning of 2021, approximately four million people, or 1.2 percent of the U.S. population, had been vaccinated, falling far short of projected time lines. By contrast, Israel, admittedly a much smaller country, had vaccinated approximately 10 percent of its population. Why

The Turning Point. Michael D. Stein and Sandro Galea, Oxford University Press.
© Oxford University Press 2024. DOI: 10.1093/oso/9780197749685.003.0001

did the United States, leading the world throughout 2020 in vaccine manufacturing, all of a sudden find itself playing catch-up in actually vaccinating its population and reopening the country? The issue was not supply. The U.S. government had bought hundreds of millions of vaccine doses, enough to vaccinate most of the population, and the pharmaceutical companies were delivering. Nor was the issue demand. It was, rather, our capacity to get vaccines to the people who were eagerly awaiting them.

Action on vaccination was delegated to the states, leaving to each the responsibility of prioritizing who got vaccinated and, as importantly, how the vaccine was delivered. This decentralization created room for innovation in delivery. West Virginia, for example, became the first state to vaccinate residents of all its nursing homes—hot spots throughout the pandemic—through a partnership with pharmacies. But some state rollouts were marked by confusion and poor execution. Each day of delay added to the tally of infections and deaths. It is one thing to have well-thought-out plans for vaccine delivery prioritization. It is another thing to actually operationalize these plans, to get the vaccines to the population.

Mass vaccination efforts live and die on the strength of the granular details of execution: who does what, when they do it, and how, and whether they are supported by resources adequate to their task. It was on us, collectively, to pursue the execution of vaccination with as much rigor as we pursued planning. It was on us to train a generation of students to be expert in implementation, to see *doing* as a task as noble as *thinking*. Vaccination, of course, accelerated in the months after its initial rollout, but it continued to fall frustratingly short of where we imagined it could be. Our sentinel success of the pandemic era—vaccination—ultimately never lived up to its promise because we fell short when it came to the practical work of making our plans a reality. Doing better next time means prioritizing our engagement with the practical, to achieve a balance between our aspirations and our operations.

2

NEXT TIME, TESTING FIRST

In 2020, biomedical science had an astounding, unprecedented year. Two vaccines were developed for a new coronavirus in less than 12 months. An entirely new mRNA technology proved sound. Clinical trials of several therapeutics were completed, and the drugs were approved for use with patients. Less impressive, readily accessible COVID-19 testing, and an at-home test with no delay in results, became available only in the final weeks of 2020. That testing arrived so late in the year, after the United States had experienced a per capita rate of testing far lower than that of most other high-income countries, was one of the great public health disappointments of the pandemic.

This failure was particularly disappointing when we compare the performance of the United States with that of other countries. Other countries that lacked rapid home testing were nevertheless able to make better use of the medically supervised, slower, "gold standard" COVID-19 tests than the United States. Asian countries had widely available testing machines and systems to evaluate which locations had excess capacity. With their smaller numbers of infections, contact tracing, isolation, and quarantine proved successful for disease control. These measures were also culturally acceptable to an extent they never were in the United States.

The Turning Point. Michael D. Stein and Sandro Galea, Oxford University Press.
© Oxford University Press 2024. DOI: 10.1093/oso/9780197749685.003.0002

Instead, we left each state mostly to its own devices—literally. State after state had insufficient supplies and inadequate testing capacity. For a disease such as COVID-19, where someone without symptoms can infect others, regular testing is critical, and an accurate, inexpensive, nonprescription, self-administered, quick-answer, home-based test would have been our best chance of limiting the spread of the disease, allowing infected individuals to learn their status sooner and avoid infecting others.

One public health lesson for the next pandemic is that spending federal dollars to help develop at-home self-diagnostic tests from the start will save lives. The public prefers convenience and self-determination. Thus, our best hope of infection control will be a simple test (a swab of the nose or mouth) that provides results in minutes and detects the early part of the disease when people are most infectious. And we need it to be widely available and affordable, with an easy reporting system so that local health departments can be informed of positive results. During COVID-19, the federal government spent tens of billions of dollars researching and purchasing vaccines, and to good effect. Next time, let's do the same for testing, and start early.

THE IRREPLACEABLE
PUBLIC SECTOR

At the start of his term, President Biden launched unprecedented, large-scale efforts to rebuild national infrastructure and to implement programs to support those most affected
by the COVID-19 pandemic. This came as a dramatic contrast
with his predecessor, whose efforts were much more in line with
Republican administrations dating back to President Reagan,
aiming to reduce the size of government and to limit the scope
of the public sector as much as possible. In the wake of a global
pandemic that froze the world's normal activities and had already
killed 400,000 Americans, the return to an engaged, muscular
public sector was a welcome shift in early 2021. From the point of
view of the decision-making that was needed to support health,
greater engagement of the public sector was not only welcome but
also essential, both to mitigate the pandemic and to help prevent
a future one.

In March 2021, President Biden introduced his "Build Back
Better" proposal, a $2.3 trillion once-in-a-generation investment,
the largest government intervention since the 1960s. To be spread
over eight years, this proposal tackled "infrastructure"—roads,
bridges, and utilities—and was not framed as an effort to address

The Turning Point. Michael D. Stein and Sandro Galea, Oxford University Press.
© Oxford University Press 2024. DOI: 10.1093/oso/9780197749685.003.0003

the nation's health. But in meaningful ways, health was at the heart of "Build Back Better." The proposal addressed many of the drivers of health that shape the world in which COVID-19 emerged. By attending to child care ($25 billion), affordable housing ($213 billion), home care for seniors ($400 billion), public transportation, and even the removal of all lead water pipes in the country, the legislation took on the conditions and structures that create poor health. All these efforts could have improved the situations of millions and addressed the vulnerabilities that COVID-19 exposed.

In the end, much of what Biden proposed did not pass, and it was the states, not Congress or the president, that decided where most of any federal infrastructure funds were spent. We leave it to others to argue about the political merits of President Biden's approach. One could argue that the spread of funds was too broad even for the expansive scope of infrastructure. There is also a healthy debate to be had over the extent to which ambitious federal spending may help create the conditions for inflation, of the type we later saw in the United States. Nevertheless, the immediate outcome of "Build Back Better" would almost certainly have been that citizens' quality of life would have improved. Jobs would have been created, and some of the work that is too costly or unprofitable for the private sector to do—for example, water and sewer system repair— would have been accomplished, with direct benefits for health.

For too long, we have neglected the structural drivers of poor health. These include the foundational challenges that large-scale federal initiatives could address. The COVID-19 moment helped reveal just how deeply rooted these challenges are. It also showed us the key role the public sector can play in strengthening the foundations of the public's health.

4

HOLDING OUR BREATH

On February 24, 2020, the first documented U.S. case of community transmission of COVID-19 was reported from a specimen collected by the Seattle Flu Study. The Seattle Flu Study was designed as a surveillance of persons reporting respiratory symptoms. In a normal year, it detects high rates of influenza, particularly during winter months—most years, influenza sickens hundreds of thousands of Americans and kills 30,000–50,000. However, 2020 was anything but a normal year. Even as the surveillance system was picking up COVID-19 cases, of the thousands of nasal swabs the research team had analyzed, an extraordinarily low number tested positive for influenza.

COVID-19, like influenza, is a virus that moves through the air. We might have expected that with so much COVID-19 around, flu would have been a fellow traveler, likewise infecting millions of Americans. But the only virus that had a successfully infectious year in 2020 was COVID-19. Other respiratory viruses were rarer too, such as respiratory syncytial virus (RSV), parainfluenza, and even other coronaviruses that cause common colds. It was not easy to find people with coughs, running noses, and fevers—symptoms typical during the winter months—who were not singularly infected with COVID-19.

The Turning Point. Michael D. Stein and Sandro Galea, Oxford University Press.
© Oxford University Press 2024. DOI: 10.1093/oso/9780197749685.003.0004

Why? Perhaps the behavioral changes triggered by COVID-19—masking, handwashing, physical distancing—had made a difference. With businesses and offices shut, with sick leaves taken more seriously, with schools and day care sites closed, with an immobilized population, there was less social interaction, which also may have helped decrease illness rates. Influenza vaccination rates throughout the country were a bit higher but probably not enough to explain the drop in what had historically been our most lethal infectious disease. This suggests that COVID-19 really was far easier to catch than more common respiratory illnesses.

It is worth noting that other respiratory diseases re-emerged during the so-called tripledemic of fall 2022, when COVID-19, flu, and RSV posed a threat to health while masks were used far less and gatherings were more common. A spike in RSV may have been attributable, in part, to lack of exposure among children during lockdowns, when RSV rates were low. If this was, in fact, the case, it reflects the complicated nature of infectious disease and how lockdowns can sometimes help us defer but not entirely avoid infectious threats.

What did we learn, then, about respiratory illness during a pandemic? First, we learned public health measures work—not only for COVID-19 but also for influenza and other common respiratory illnesses. At the same time, the effects of these measures are not without costs and complexities, as in the case of RSV. Second, we learned that surveillance, one of the core activities of public health, works. Influenza surveillance centers already exist throughout the world and, along with local studies such as that in Seattle, were scouting for COVID-19 as it entered its second year among humans. Third, new vaccine technologies will matter when influenza recurs. In the past, flu vaccines took half a year to develop and manufacture; the RNA-based COVID-19 shots are easier and faster to update and may make us nimbler in adjusting vaccine ingredients to novel influenza strains that arise and from which we need protection. Can we embed these lessons in our approach to respiratory disease going forward? If we do, this may be one of the positive legacies of this COVID-19 moment.

5

THE CHALLENGE
OF ADDRESSING
MULTIPLE CRISES

The COVID-19 moment was, in fact, many moments. It was the time of a pandemic, but it was also the time of other, intersecting challenges, all of which had implications for health. Well into the pandemic, on February 24, 2022, Russia invaded Ukraine, creating a level of conflict not seen in Europe since World War II. The war brought untold suffering to the people of Ukraine and raised the specter of nuclear war, as Russia threatened to escalate the conflict and the United States committed to supporting Ukraine against aggression.

War is always a catastrophe for health, particularly for the civilian populations that are inevitably caught in the crossfire. Wars can also lead to mass migration as populations flee conflict zones, creating unique challenges for the health of migrants and their communities. In the atomic age, conflict—or even just the possibility of conflict—between nuclear-armed nations poses a threat to every life on earth. To be concerned with the public's health, then, is to be concerned with war—with preventing it when possible and with mitigating its effects when not. A war as blatantly

The Turning Point. Michael D. Stein and Sandro Galea, Oxford University Press.
© Oxford University Press 2024. DOI: 10.1093/oso/9780197749685.003.0005

unjust as Russia's war on Ukraine adds urgency to this imperative. Such aggression is not just a violation of the health of populations (in Ukraine, COVID-19 care was certainly deprioritized after the invasion) and the territorial integrity of a country. It is a violation of progress itself, of our collective hope for a future that is more humane, more decent than our past. The work of public health is the work of creating such a future.

In addition to the context of the war in Ukraine, the pandemic unfolded in the context of a threat arguably just as existential as that of global war: climate change. The earth is one degree hotter than it was during the Industrial Revolution. This may not seem like much, but it has been enough to lengthen our fire season and burn 20 percent of Australia's forests in one summer, to make our days the hottest in recorded history, and to have bleached 90 percent of the Great Barrier Reef. Climate change has expanded the range and prevalence of some infectious diseases, including Lyme disease and West Nile virus in the United States. Deforestation, which harms our atmosphere, has brought more wild animals (and zoonotic illness) into contact with humans.

And the world is not going to get cooler. Current estimates predict a two degree rise by the 2030s, three degrees by 2050; if the arctic permafrost thaws or tropical rainforests are razed, this timing could accelerate. Two degrees is not twice as bad as one degree; damage and displacement will be exponential, not linear. At two degrees higher, most East Coast residents will need sea walls to maintain their homes, at the cost of approximately $1 million per resident. No one will want to pay this.

The challenge of addressing overlapping crises seems to suggest an obvious question: What do we address first? The intersecting threats of the early 2020s—war, climate, and COVID-19—all posed significant challenges for health. We have a responsibility to engage with threats to the public's health, but how do we weigh the moral burden of doing so in a context of finite time and resources? The answer lies in challenging the terms of the question. Rather than address multiple crises as discrete issues, we need to become better at seeing the areas where they intersect and then addressing them at the level of this complexity. War, climate, and COVID-19 are all to some extent emergent properties of injustice, misguided collective priorities, and an unwillingness to forthrightly address long-festering problems. Addressing such challenges—the fundamental drivers of so much poor health—could help us make a positive difference on many fronts at once.

6

THE INVISIBLE MENTAL HEALTH BURDENS OF A PANDEMIC

When COVID-19 emerged as a global pandemic at the beginning of 2020, it soon dominated global headlines, as country after country tried to manage the increased burden of infection and the attendant rise in hospitalizations and deaths. As countries struggled to contain the pandemic, efforts to social distance and limit interpersonal contact shut down businesses and plunged the global economy into a recession. Time and again, as the pandemic appeared to recede, it resurged, delivering a fresh wave of increased cases and varying degrees of restrictions on our daily activities, which in turn had profound effects on our inner lives.

The fear of the pandemic, the economic downturn, the shutdown of schools, and the disruption of everyday life constituted a perfect storm for increasing poor mental health nationally and globally. Mental health is particularly responsive to stressful conditions. Previous large-scale traumatic events have taught us that there is an uptick in persons reporting common mood and anxiety disorders, notably depression and post-traumatic stress

The Turning Point. Michael D. Stein and Sandro Galea, Oxford University Press.
© Oxford University Press 2024. DOI: 10.1093/oso/9780197749685.003.0006

disorder, after such events. COVID-19 presented a particularly challenging set of circumstances for mental health. Fear of infection was a traumatic influence that would have been bad enough for mental health on its own. Even worse was its coupling with the sudden rise in unemployment and the large-scale civil unrest that hit the United States in the summer of 2020.

Following the emergence of multiple, intersecting national traumas, study after study showed that the burden of mood and anxiety disorders increased up to threefold over baseline during the COVID-19 pandemic and that this upturn was geographically widespread. Although this may not have been surprising, what followed was. As COVID-19 continued, so did the high rates of poor mental health a year into the pandemic. And data started to emerge about the concomitant behavioral health challenges that are frequently comorbid with poor mental health. Smoking rates increased in some groups, as did use of alcohol. Most dramatically, the number of fatal drug overdose deaths soared, with more than 100,000 people dying in the first 12 months of the pandemic, representing a 30 percent increase over the prior 12 months, which was already at a historic high.

As a pandemic recedes, we may expect that, for many, the heightened symptoms of depression and anxiety will also resolve. But the burden of the poor mental health that emerges from pandemic moments may last a lifetime. Having had prior mental illness is the best documented risk factor for future mental illness, meaning that the baseline risk for future poor mental health can be elevated for a generation in the wake of a pandemic such as COVID-19. The costs of increased substance use may be felt in the accompanying chronic disease burden a pandemic-affected cohort may face in the decades after a contagion strikes. Ultimately, the invisible mental health burden may affect as many, if not more, lives than a virus itself touches directly. This calls for a rigorous look at the services that we make available to help mitigate poor mental health in the decades ahead and for carefully weighing the price we pay in poor mental health as we implement efforts to control infectious disease outbreaks in the future.

7

PANDEMIC AND PRISONS

Throughout the pandemic, we saw how COVID-19 was worsened by existing problems that had long been present. These problems—from racism to economic inequality and political dysfunction—made us vulnerable to contagion, and they continue to do so.

As the pandemic unfolded, it became clear that prisons represented one of these problems, as part of a status quo driving poorer health. Prisons have long played a role in keeping the United States less healthy than it could be. The incarceration rate in the United States is higher than in any other country in the world, and it is approximately five times higher than the median rate worldwide. The health consequences of incarceration are legion. Disability-adjusted life year rates linked to incarceration are more than double those attributed to other conditions commonly experienced by the general population. Death rates are high and are the result of overcrowding, inadequate mental health care, lousy sanitation, freezing temperatures, and delayed medical treatments. Half of prison suicides result from solitary confinement.

The burdens of incarceration are deeply and unevenly felt. African Americans are incarcerated at five times the rate of White

The Turning Point. Michael D. Stein and Sandro Galea, Oxford University Press.
© Oxford University Press 2024. DOI: 10.1093/oso/9780197749685.003.0007

Americans. Nearly half of all Black women have a family member in prison. One in three Black men born today will end up in the correctional system at some point. The bias against people of color is operationalized at many levels: through police arresting minorities at higher rates than Whites and through prosecutors charging them more often and more severely, leading to longer sentences.

Given this context, it is little surprise that COVID-19 posed a particular challenge to the populations of prisons and jails. Social distancing and quarantines were nearly impossible in such settings—the jail on Rikers Island, for example, had one toilet for every 29 people. The COVID-19 case rate was four times higher in state and federal prisons than in the general population—and twice as deadly. Despite reductions in state prison populations (mostly due to decreased admissions over 2021), prisons and jails were the sites of most large, single-site outbreaks of COVID-19. Yet only 10 states explicitly put incarcerated people in phase one of vaccine distribution at the start of the vaccination rollout, and eight states did not list them in any phase of vaccine distribution.

Can anything mitigate the challenge incarceration poses to public health? The experience of a pandemic makes the question even more urgent, and the answer, fortunately, is yes. Centrally, the reallocation of funds from policing and incarceration to the work of public health—violence prevention programs, community mental health care, housing, and education—may reduce prison populations. We should not miss this opportunity to address the challenge of incarceration and mitigate our country's many failures on this issue. Addressing incarceration can also help model the kind of engagement necessary for addressing other pre-existing problems that keep us vulnerable to sickness, toward shaping a healthier context in which pandemics are less likely to take hold.

8

THE NECESSITY OF
SPEAKING WITH CARE

In Fyodor Dostoevsky's novel, *The Brothers Karamazov*, one of the titular brothers, Ivan Karamazov, struggles with a crisis of faith—or, rather, lack of faith. Ivan cannot accept the existence of a God who would allow so much suffering in the world. Because he cannot reason himself into believing in a loving God, he cannot believe in a basis for objective morality, his arguments amounting to the famous phrase that "If there is no God, everything is permitted." Throughout the novel, Ivan shares his theories with various characters, speaking eloquently and authoritatively. Yet his story ends in madness after it is revealed that Smerdyakov, his father's servant, found his arguments a bit too convincing and acted on them by murdering and robbing Ivan's father, Fyodor Pavlovich. The real-world effects of Ivan's philosophy prove too much, and at the novel's conclusion he is in a state of mental illness, his fate unclear.

During COVID-19, public health often found itself speaking with the didactic confidence of Ivan. We spoke—to policymakers, to the public, and on social media—of the need for an aggressive strategy of lockdowns, masking, and vaccination. Some voices in our field argued that the threat of the virus was so acute that

The Turning Point. Michael D. Stein and Sandro Galea, Oxford University Press.

nothing less than a zero-COVID strategy would do. Like the atheist who reasons themself out of belief in God, we could be dismissive of those who did not share our conclusions, meeting with hostility those arguing for a more measured approach to the crisis.

We were able to speak too assertively because, in our heart of hearts, we perhaps did not really think that the effects of the prolonged lockdowns required to achieve zero-COVID would ever come to pass. Just as Ivan was able, for a time, to avoid being confronted with what his philosophy could lead to if carried to its logical conclusion, public health authorities could make pronouncements in the realm of theory without having to face the practical consequences of our words. We did not always consider that words have a life of their own and we can never be sure who is listening or how our words will be interpreted.

As it turned out during COVID-19, China, like Smerdyakov, was listening. And China was all too willing to implement an authoritarian approach to the pandemic. Its pursuit of zero-COVID showed us what our lines of reasoning can look like when actually carried out at scale, with the full force of government backing them up. What we saw was, in many ways, as horrible as what Ivan saw in the actions of Smerdyakov. Crackdowns, repression, and a halting of anything resembling normal life characterized China's draconian approach to the pandemic. Its pursuit of zero-COVID yielded some initial success, but at the cost of the freedom of tens of millions. The cruelty of this approach was reflected in an apartment fire in which COVID-19 restrictions may have prevented first responders from getting to the blaze, which killed 10 people. Eventually, protests motivated a lifting of restrictions, but not until after months of suffering, much of it justified in the name of public health.

It would, of course, be unfair to blame the worst aspects of the Chinese approach to COVID-19 entirely on public health. China has a long history of human rights violations, including mass surveillance and the ongoing persecution of its Uyghur population. However, it is also true that China's zero-COVID approach aligned with what many in public health called for during the pandemic.

Public health has a responsibility to weigh its words carefully and to speak out when we see abuses being committed in our name. At this turning point moment, the voice of public health carries farther than ever, amplified by social media, our engagement with policymakers, and the experience of a pandemic that turned the world to us as sources of expertise. We should never forget that many are listening and that some may be willing, and able, to use our recommendations to justify actions that harm others. We should tread softly, then, speaking with humility and avoiding an overly confident tone that suggests we are more certain than we are.

9

HEALTH BEHAVIOR

The conditions of where we live, work, and play, our money and our resources, deeply shape our health. But how, exactly? Through a variety of mechanisms, one of which is, unquestionably, by affecting our behavior. If I am living in a dangerous, unwalkable neighborhood, for example, I am less likely to exercise and more likely to suffer from obesity and attendant heart disease. So, behavior is closely linked to the world around us. For this reason, it should be central to our efforts to improve the health of populations.

This is never clearer than during a pandemic. Differential early burden of COVID-19 was driven in no small part by changes in behavior. As those with resources were able to shift rapidly to working from home, they had lower risk of acquiring COVID-19, and subsequent lower burden of infection and death from the pandemic. Yet as COVID-19 progressed, prolonged social isolation became associated with harmful behaviors, including the use of substances, leading to a surge of poor health.

That we were unable to mitigate the drivers of risky health behaviors during COVID-19 highlights a fundamental problem we have with health behaviors: They are influenced by the world around us, and they are difficult to change. Although public health

The Turning Point. Michael D. Stein and Sandro Galea, Oxford University Press.
© Oxford University Press 2024. DOI: 10.1093/oso/9780197749685.003.0009

is built on success stories such as reducing smoking or promoting seat belt wearing, these changes took decades, further emphasizing how difficult it is to effectively change behaviors around health. And although we often imagine that having adequate risk information at hand will lead us to make different behavioral choices, studies repeatedly have shown this not to be the case.

What might we learn from the pandemic experience that can nudge us toward better health behaviors? Two points suggest a way forward.

First, it is imperative that we bear in mind that context shapes health behaviors. For example, it is not a surprise that millions of people staying at home and the social isolation which goes with that are associated with greater substance misuse and attendant drug overdose. Such observations should be part of our calculus when we are creating policies to change context to better support health.

Second, health behaviors are often driven by broad social phenomena. It is likely, for example, that the move to stay indoors during a pandemic has as much to do with fear of a disease as it does with any specific stay-at-home orders. This suggests that the tools for changing behavior should extend well beyond the individual, to fundamentally address our cultural norms.

These observations do not solve all of our problems with health behaviors. Our behaviors remain difficult to change and always will. But these points do perhaps sharpen our thinking about the importance of engaging with context in supporting healthier behaviors, respecting the role the world in which we live plays in how we navigate each day.

10

THE CARING INFRASTRUCTURE

COVID-19 exposed social problems that existed long before the pandemic struck. For one, the virus exacerbated long-ignored challenges we faced in caring for the elderly, the disabled, and younger children. Nursing homes became centers of infection and death during the pandemic. Group homes, day care, and home care services for the disabled and elderly disappeared. Schools closed. Caregivers rose to the top of the list of our most essential workers. As this workforce faced risk, sickness among caregivers further weakened the substructure holding up our shaky economy.

These challenges strained a system already under stress. Before the pandemic struck, backlogs for home- and community-based care were impossibly long for hundreds of thousands of people. At that time, inadequate services primarily burdened low-income Americans who had to rely on government-subsidized caregiving. During COVID-19, the shortage became an issue for everyone. Fifty-three million family members were already providing most of the care for vulnerable seniors and people with disabilities before the pandemic. With the emergence of COVID-19, as caregiving shortages became rampant, the burden of caregiving fell to

The Turning Point. Michael D. Stein and Sandro Galea, Oxford University Press.
© Oxford University Press 2024. DOI: 10.1093/oso/9780197749685.003.0010

everyone, making it difficult for families with two working adults to juggle caregiving responsibilities. Without care options, many adults, most often women, left the workforce.

Essential work, as is now abundantly understood, has historically been underpaid. COVID-19 exposed this for all to see. Caregivers, such as nursing assistants and home health and personal care aides, earn on average $12 an hour. Most are women of color; approximately one-third of those working for agencies do not receive health insurance from their employers.

Pre-COVID-19, our system of care was broken, unfixed by the market economy. In large part, this challenge was created by lack of investment in caregiving as a public good. We need a larger, better paid, better trained workforce of caregivers. Such a workforce will take years to organize, supported by political will. The pandemic changed our politics, but can government spending really expand services, eliminate waiting lists, and increase salaries? We shall see.

11

DOES TODAY MATTER MORE
THAN TOMORROW?

COVID-19 showed us that the present can be, at times, overwhelming. At the start of the pandemic, in the first terrifying
months of a disease that we did not understand, it was appropriate
that we invested every bit of our effort in mitigating the immediate
threat we faced. As we learned more about the disease, however—
and improved our capacity to prevent and treat it—a debate
emerged about the extent to which our earlier efforts to slow the
spread of the virus were still worth the trade-offs they entailed. We
found ourselves asking, at what point does supporting health in
the present yield to the importance of laying the groundwork for
a healthier future?

There are several ways we can approach this question.
Economists approach it through time discounting—the study of
how the value of rewards is shaped by their temporal proximity.
Benefits that accrue in the present tend to matter more than those
that may accrue in the future, losing value the more distant they
become from the present moment, simply because, all things
being equal, we put more value on the bird in the hand. There are,
of course, alternative perspectives. If we prioritize the needs of
future generations—as in the case, for example, of a parent who

The Turning Point. Michael D. Stein and Sandro Galea, Oxford University Press.
© Oxford University Press 2024. DOI: 10.1093/oso/9780197749685.003.0011

invests their money into college funds for their children rather than buying a new car—we are valuing the future more than the present.

The pandemic showed us how an overinvestment in the present can cause us to lose sight of challenges that will affect our health in the long term. Data emerged about excess mortality during the COVID-19 period—mortality caused by a range of other diseases, from Alzheimer's to heart disease. These deaths were likely due to a combination of an overstressed and underresourced health care system dealing with an influx of hospitalizations, and infectious disease precautions and changes in behavior influenced by fear of COVID-19. We also know that the social isolation that accompanied COVID-19 mitigation efforts was linked to a dramatic increase in poor mental health, the consequences of which remain with us.

The choice between the needs of today and tomorrow, between the urgent and the important, is resonant in health. We are charged with generating health for as many people as possible throughout their life course. This requires us to focus on the present, but also to look beyond the present to focus on the future. The balance of the urgent and the important requires constant recalibration. During COVID-19, we were perhaps too slow at thinking about tomorrow as we engaged with the urgencies of today.

12

TELLING DIFFERENT STORIES
WITH THE SAME DATA

Measuring our successes in creating healthy populations is, in large part, a matter of the data we choose to emphasize in the story we tell about our health. By one metric, for example, the United States is doing quite well in its pursuit of health. Compared to most of the world—indeed, compared to most of human history—we enjoy fantastic health, supported by a standard of living that is truly enviable. These data let us tell a story about our health that is broadly optimistic about the path we are on. However, when compared to peer countries—nations with a standard of living comparable to ours—our health is mediocre. The United States spends far more on health care than any of its peer high-income countries. Yet we have lower life expectancy at birth than our peers. One story of our health these data tell is that we are not getting a good return on our health investment. But we also perform better than almost all of our peer countries when it comes to supporting the health of persons older than age 75 years—when health care becomes most important. A story can then be told that we value our health throughout the life course

The Turning Point. Michael D. Stein and Sandro Galea, Oxford University Press.
© Oxford University Press 2024. DOI: 10.1093/oso/9780197749685.003.0012

and that we spend accordingly, prolonging life, aligned with our national values.

The limited role data play in shaping the stories we tell ourselves about our health was clear during COVID-19. We struggled initially with what our goalposts should be, whether we considered success primarily a matter of having lower cases or fewer deaths. This choice shaped how well we considered ourselves to be doing at any given moment during the pandemic. This accounts for why there was such controversy, even within public health, about which way the winds were blowing during the pandemic and what course to take in the face of an evolving threat.

Our view of COVID-19 data was also shaped by the premium we placed on health equity. Early rapid success in vaccination—the single most effective means of mitigating viral spread—was accompanied by racial/ethnic gaps in vaccination. In most states, White people received a higher share of vaccinations compared with their share of cases, widening racial gaps when it came to COVID-19 risk. Was early vaccination achievement then a success, or was it a failure? And the vaccines themselves remained extraordinarily effective even as the more transmissible delta variant swept the country. Among fully vaccinated people, the reinfection rate was less than 1 percent; fewer than 0.004 percent needed hospitalization, and fewer than 0.001 percent died from the disease. Yet concern about the delta variant dramatically changed the public perception of our success in mitigating COVID-19 in the summer of 2021, leading many to believe vaccines made little difference.

All of this teaches us that the same data can become the foundation of very different stories. As such, a reliance on data alone to shape the narratives that guide our policymaking is a mistake. It teaches us that those who engage in science have a collective responsibility to generate data but also to help mold the stories that shape the public conversation that ultimately informs politics and policies.

13

HOW OUR EXPECTATIONS SHAPE OUR PERCEPTIONS OF REALITY

In 2021, Japan hosted the 2020 Summer Olympics, staged that year due to a year-long COVID-19 delay. Japan, by any number of metrics, did extraordinarily well at the games, coming in third in the gold medal count, handily outperforming other traditionally successful Olympic powerhouses. Yet, despite this success, many Japanese athletes felt compelled to deliver tearful apologies at their "failures" on winning silver medals.

The curious case of Japanese regret in a moment of ostensible triumph can only be explained when we remember that data (in this case, the medal type and count) are simply one input that shapes our understanding of meaning and truth. The Olympics were held amid substantial local controversy as Japan faced a surge in its COVID-19 cases. This made for added pressure on the host country to do well, so much so that anything short of gold was viewed as a failure. This was a dramatic reminder of the powerful role that our expectation of success plays in our perception of that very success.

The Turning Point. Michael D. Stein and Sandro Galea, Oxford University Press.
© Oxford University Press 2024. DOI: 10.1093/oso/9780197749685.003.0013

Consider the COVID-19 summer of 2021 in the United States. What started as a season of optimism, with President Biden declaring a summer of freedom with the COVID-19 vaccine, quickly turned sour when, less than a month later, a majority of Americans again thought that the worst of the pandemic was ahead of them rather than behind them. The rise of the delta variant fueled a dramatic change in American public perception as the United States started experiencing an increase in COVID-19 cases which had been waning over the earlier months of summer. But the delta variant was not doing anything that was unanticipated. It was driving viral spread among those who were unvaccinated, with a clear inverse correlation between state-level vaccination rates and new COVID-19 infections. Critically, those who had received the vaccine had a very low risk of reacquiring COVID-19 and were at even lower risk of being hospitalized or dying from the virus. In addition, we had a precedent for how we were going to do with the delta variant, as the United Kingdom preceded the United States by about a month in its epidemic curve and readily showed that we could expect a waxing—and then a waning—of new infections, principally among the unvaccinated in the United States.

The rise of the delta variant shaped our experience of COVID-19 in the United States during the summer of 2021 in large part because after the third wave of COVID-19 in the spring of 2021, our national expectation was that the worst was over. But stories about "breakthrough" infections returned COVID-19 to the headlines, displacing any sense we may have had that we were in a dramatically different phase of the pandemic—although we were. We entered the summer of 2021 expecting gold and instead got silver. This was intolerable to us.

All of this suggests the importance of managing expectations, particularly during acute health crises. It matters little how many "medals" we win as a country—what might matter more is whether we win more, or less, than we expected. Similarly, COVID-19 taught us that baseline expectation setting—and an awareness of the role that expectation plays in our own psychology—is critical for health if we are to be reasonably grounded in a data-informed reality. We want to make health decisions that are informed neither by unfounded exuberance nor by irrational malaise and to avoid the unwarranted defeatism that can arise when we devalue silver medals.

14

CAN CONTACT TRACING WORK HERE?

One of the disappointments in our response to the pandemic was the limited ability of our contact tracing—one of the fundamental activities of public health during an infectious disease outbreak—to control COVID-19 transmission. In the United States, our poor performance in this area was in marked contrast to other countries. Hong Kong and Singapore, for example, initially contained their outbreaks by deploying thousands of public health workers to track down every person with a newly positive test, figure out with whom they had been in contact, and quickly get those people into quarantine. The United States did not.

Why did we do so poorly compared to other countries? The U.S. public health system faced three challenges in its attempt to make contact tracing work. First, we had inadequate COVID-19 testing early on: We could not identify all positive cases. The testing system failed, with long waits to get tests and then more waiting for results. Without being able to readily identify and test those who had been in contact with an infected person, the chain of infection continued. By the time testing was readily available, rapid, and mostly free, the number of people infected far outstripped the supply of contact tracers.

The Turning Point. Michael D. Stein and Sandro Galea, Oxford University Press.
© Oxford University Press 2024. DOI: 10.1093/oso/9780197749685.003.0014

Even if we had accurate testing available soon after COVID-19 was identified, we still would have faced our second problem: workforce limitations. Four months into the pandemic, in May 2020, we had only a fraction of the public health workers needed to launch an effective national contact tracing effort. At that time—with only 30,000 persons having tested positive—public health experts told Congress the country needed to increase the number of contact tracing staff tenfold to 100,000 or more. Yet even in December 2020, at the peak of U.S. caseload, there were still only 70,000 contact tracers nationwide. Widespread community transmission throughout the country occurred within a few months of COVID-19's arrival; it is unclear that any number of contact tracers could have kept up. The numbers grew too big too fast.

The third challenge was the lack of trust in public health authorities and services. As reported in a Centers for Disease Control and Prevention analysis of 14 contact tracing programs from June to October 2020, "No contacts were reported for two-thirds of persons with laboratory confirmed COVID-19 because they were either not reached for an interview or were interviewed and named no contacts." In other words, citizens would not speak to contact tracing personnel.

We have learned that when the next pandemic arrives, even if we quickly create a test to identify cases, we may not be adequately prepared to perform the contact tracing necessary to control a new infection. We are not Hong Kong or Singapore, small islands with small populations. Our market economy disincentivizes inefficiency; we are unlikely to keep a workforce of already trained contact tracers waiting around for the next infectious disease to come along, so once again we would face workforce training issues. Complicating matters, distrust of government only grew stronger during the pandemic, making it less likely that a national contact tracing effort would be met by public consent. Economic and cultural forces worked against the best public health efforts with COVID-19, and only the reconsideration of these challenges will position us better next time.

15

PRESCRIPTION
AGAINST WORRY

The end of 2021 saw the arrival in the United States of the omicron variant, a highly infectious form of COVID-19 that produced another punishing wave of disruptions among the population. The sudden rise in COVID-19 cases in unvaccinated and vaccinated persons alike produced new worry about whether these infections would translate into growing numbers of hospitalizations and deaths. But as omicron spread, good news emerged. The first two oral, antiviral medications to treat symptomatic COVID-19 for those with high-risk underlying medical conditions, or who were older than age 60 years, were approved by the U.S. Food and Drug Administration. Their arrival was heralded as a game-changer. Finally, there was a simple and effective treatment that could limit the worst outcomes of infection. But the arrival of the medications once again highlighted the problems of delivering state-of-the-art care to the American population, two years into the pandemic.

The stunningly rapid creation and production of COVID-19 vaccines was also considered a game-changer, the beginning of the end of the pandemic. And indeed, the majority of Americans were vaccinated with great public and private sector effort, reducing the

The Turning Point. Michael D. Stein and Sandro Galea, Oxford University Press.
© Oxford University Press 2024. DOI: 10.1093/oso/9780197749685.003.0015

risk of serious illness. However, we fell short of vaccinating enough people to stop the pandemic, largely due to the worries that have always accompanied the introduction of a new vaccine that, in this case, were fed by widespread politicization of public health efforts.

The potential impact of the new oral medications faced a different set of hurdles. First, to use medication required proof of infection, such proof required testing as confirmation, and testing remained hard to come by at the start of 2022. The United States never took seriously the notion that frequent COVID-19 testing was critical to managing the pandemic and continued to underinvest in testing two years into the crisis. At the same time as these revolutionary drugs were being rolled out, tests were still not widely available and take-home versions were expensive, affordable to only a few.

Second and relatedly, the benefits of COVID-19 medication depended on treatment starting within three to five days of diagnosis, which meant recognizing symptoms (which during winter months could be due to other viruses), performing a confirmatory test, and then finding a medical provider to explain risks and benefits and offer a prescription.

Third, approximately 30 million Americans having no medical insurance and tens of millions more having inadequate insurance meant these citizens would have to pay for medical appointments as well as for the new medications. Unlike masks, quarantines, and even vaccines, these medications required interaction with our health care system, which once again exposed our long-standing challenges with equitable access to care.

Finally, until these medications were tested across tens of thousands of patients, the full side effect profiles remained uncertain and we faced the prospect of newly detected side effects that would be overblown in media reports, derailing use over the first few months of the new drugs' rollout.

These challenges were a reminder that dealing with a pandemic does not happen in a vacuum. The success or failure of any strategy, no matter how high tech or impressive, depends on the underlying structure of the health system tasked with delivering it, on whether the population would be willing to accept it, and on the many other details that decide whether we are positioned for success. To beat back a pandemic, we need to address these foundational challenges *before* the pandemic ever hits. This may be the most important COVID-19 lesson of all.

SECTION 2

STORY

HEALTH is fundamentally a story. This story is about much more than just doctors and medicines—it is about the socioeconomic conditions in which we live. How we tell the story of these conditions will shape how well we can leverage this turning point into a future where pandemics can no longer take hold.

16

POLITICAL DECISIONS
AND SCIENCE

In early 2021, *The Boston Globe* ran a story titled "After Baker relaxes some pandemic restrictions, epidemiologists urge caution." The article noted that, citing an improvement in the pandemic curve, Massachusetts Governor Charlie Baker announced he would relax rules that required many restaurants to close at 9:30 p.m. The article went on to quote several experts about this, all of whom warned that this adjustment came too soon. Tellingly, one of the experts quoted was "not privy to all the data the Baker administration has and acknowledged that there are economic and psychological factors to consider when it comes to assessing restrictions."

These factors are indeed core to the choices we make about health. Fundamentally, decisions about health—including about COVID-19—are political decisions. They should take into account the science, but they should also balance a range of other considerations. As news outlets were reporting on hesitance among some health authorities to lift pandemic restrictions, there were also stories about surges in suicides among school-age

The Turning Point. Michael D. Stein and Sandro Galea, Oxford University Press.
© Oxford University Press 2024. DOI: 10.1093/oso/9780197749685.003.0016

children in Las Vegas, which resulted in school reopening, a scenario long anticipated by the Centers for Disease Control and Prevention. Surely such reports should be a consideration in decisions to maintain or relax restrictions during a pandemic.

Experts quoted by *The Boston Globe* went on to say that they were willing to "endure continued restrictions in January and February even though it stinks, in order to have a better May, June, and July." It may well be that a particular expert preferred to endure restrictions in January and February, but all evidence was that the governor balanced the costs of these restrictions—economic, social, and psychological—with the costs of no longer maintaining them. What did it then mean that experts were lined up by a prominent newspaper for a story that essentially aimed to undercut the complex balance that a governor—who by all accounts acted responsibly and prudently for the duration of the pandemic—was trying to strike in determining appropriate ways to handle the pandemic? Did such a story serve the public good?

Although epidemiologists have long been widely respected within public health, providing the quantitative heart of much of population health science, the field had never quite been in the public eye as it was during COVID-19. Such a rise in visibility, and the growing reliance of policymaking on the opinion of scientific experts, comes with power—the power to influence decisions and to change daily life for millions of Americans.

When the engagement of population health scientists with the media was more infrequent, and perhaps less consequential, experts enjoyed the luxury of casual assertion without much fear that it might tip the balance of action. When that is no longer the case, our caution in what we say, and in when we say it, should increase commensurately. The public weighs our words, as do politicians, with significant effects on the lives of many. It is important that we wield this influence responsibly, by considering the full range of factors that should influence decision-making around health.

17

SHOULD WE BE MORE UPSET BY THIS?

The world was upended during 2020 by COVID-19. As we struggled with the pandemic, much of life as we knew it ground to a halt. We watched case counts rise, anguished over severe cases . . . and waited for a vaccine. We started talking about the potential for a vaccine as early as March 2020, giving us at least eight months of lead time to be ready to implement a program of mass immunization once the vaccines were approved.

Vaccines finally arrived in December 2020, yet this program, for the most part, did not materialize. And we all fretted and wrung our hands in frustration. But were we as upset as we should have been? After all, this was a vaccine rollout that we *knew* was going to be needed and that we *knew* would be happening soon enough. Yet it was subpar at best, botched at worst. With this in mind, we probably should have been even more upset at our failure and called loudly for reform of the vaccine rollout process. Why did this not happen? Why was there little vaccine activism, to focus attention on our shortcomings and urge us to do better next time?

First, it was not at all obvious that there was a group that could have taken the lead on galvanizing our ire during the COVID-19 moment. Those at highest risk of COVID-19—the elderly, those

The Turning Point. Michael D. Stein and Sandro Galea, Oxford University Press.
© Oxford University Press 2024. DOI: 10.1093/oso/9780197749685.003.0017

in congregate living facilities—were much less likely to engage in activism, as opposed to other historical instances in which those most affected by societal shortcomings could effectively take to the streets.

It was also difficult to see who precisely was to blame for the COVID-19 vaccine rollout flub. The likeliest target of reproach, the president, had lied about the risks of COVID-19 from the start, and half the population had been angry at him for years for a slew of other reasons. Additional opprobrium directed his way would have been a drop in the bucket, making little difference. It is also true that the Trump administration's record on vaccines was fairly good, at least in expediting the development phase.

Other than the president, the U.S. Food and Drug Administration and the National Institutes of Health—clear targets for prior generations of activism for not producing and approving medications fast enough—had, in this case, done their jobs through the miraculous speed of vaccine creation and an approval process that moved as fast as safely possible.

In the 2020 world of conspiracies, we had no conspiracy theory to explain the slowness of the vaccine rollout. Instead, we faulted government ineptitude and negligence, which was hardly enough to galvanize a movement. It is unsatisfying to condemn bureaucracy for holdups in supply chains. Yet a better alternative did not emerge.

Perhaps by December 11, 2020, when the Pfizer vaccine was approved (the Moderna vaccine was approved on December 18), we were already exhausted as a nation. The weather was growing cold. A new administration was only approximately 30 days away. Maybe we just opted to wait, with the assumption that eventually our vaccine distribution fiasco would be resolved.

Ironically, all the visible anger and activism concerning COVID-19 had been around the "anti's"—anti-mask, anti-vaccine. The anti-activists largely worked toward the goal of personal autonomy. These activists insisted that government stay out of their lives.

The rest of us, the non-activists, mostly wanted government *in* our lives. One lesson of COVID-19 was that sometimes vigorous federal intervention on our behalf is necessary. Yet it is not enough to merely want this. We must agitate for it, or else face more failures such as the vaccine rollout. If we do not demand we do better, who will?

18

THE RESPONSIBILITY
OF EXPERTS

The COVID-19 moment created a seemingly inexhaustible demand for public health experts. For approximately two years, epidemiologists were on prime time, and all manner of public health experts appeared on television, podcasts, and social media. That the media called on such expertise to help explain the moment was very much to the good. But public health's sudden "close-up" moment also put intense focus on many who were not used to the spotlight, causing some to forget that being an expert with a public platform comes with special responsibilities.

Consider the parade of experts who tried to predict the number of people who would be infected with COVID-19. Throughout 2020, experts suggested that the final COVID-19 death tallies would be 200,000, or 2 million in the United States. All of these experts had reasoning behind their numbers. But all fundamentally knew that their estimates were based on a range of assumptions that would likely not stand the test of time. And the vast majority of estimates did not. What they did instead was spread fevered worry and seed mistrust of the scientific enterprise. After all, if scientists cannot predict the extent of the outbreak correctly, it is reasonable to wonder what else they might get wrong.

The Turning Point. Michael D. Stein and Sandro Galea, Oxford University Press.
© Oxford University Press 2024. DOI: 10.1093/oso/9780197749685.003.0018

Consider another example: the abundance of expert punditry about the need for lockdowns, which often touted the efforts of "successful" states. But time and again, the pandemic showed us that patterns of transmission were not easily predictable. States, such as California, that were one day lauded as models for prevention efforts went on the next day to face new outbreak peaks. What we did know during the pandemic was that there was substantial idiosyncrasy behind outbreak patterns, which required humility on the part of experts—a quality that turned out to be in short supply. The responsible expert approach would have been to lead with the uncertainty, making it clear we knew much less than we hoped to and that lockdown decisions were fundamentally political, with public health informing, but not dictating, actions.

Why would experts offer assertions that might falsely reassure, needlessly terrify, and generally sow confusion, undermining the very enterprise they represent? Maybe they were trying to explain complicated models that built on sophisticated approaches in the field, and doing so with mixed results. Maybe they had good intentions, aiming to be good citizens helping explain matters to the confused public. Or maybe they were just showing off.

Even if offered innocently, an "expert's" speculation that introduces reductive simplifications into the rapid metabolism of mass media spreads misinformation. It is foolhardy to offer answers that will "stick" and become headlines, without thinking through the implications of these prognostications.

The COVID-19 moment taught us that public health may not have been quite ready for the harsh glare of the global media spotlight. We need to learn from this and be ready to do better the next time around.

19

DEFINING OUR GOALPOSTS

During April 2020, the in-hospital mortality rate from COVID-19 was 19.7 percent. By November, it had declined to 9.3 percent. That was a remarkable testament to the triumph of clinical medicine in the face of a previously unknown disease. The drop in mortality was due to many factors, including the use of nonpharmacological approaches such as patient proning, the use of pharmacological therapies in hospitals such as remdesivir and steroids, and perhaps also due to lower viral loads seen in hospitalized patients because of a more universal embrace of mask-wearing. Regardless of the explanation, our handling of COVID-19 improved quickly, dramatically changing the risk of death.

But this improvement in mortality did not do very much to change our broader public narrative around COVID-19. Our impression of a new deadly disease that was to be avoided at all costs was established quickly in March 2020, and it did not budge much when the risk of the disease's feared outcome changed substantially. We saw the same dynamic a year later as the widespread introduction of vaccines provided protection for the most vulnerable—the elderly and those with underlying medical conditions—lowering mortality rates and leaving cases to be driven by younger people with much less risk of contracting severe COVID-19. Despite a

The Turning Point. Michael D. Stein and Sandro Galea, Oxford University Press.
© Oxford University Press 2024. DOI: 10.1093/oso/9780197749685.003.0019

dramatic change in disease profile due to increased vaccination, the public conversation about the state of the pandemic remained driven, largely, by fluctuating case numbers. State-by-state decisions were also informed primarily by caseload, even if these cases were milder and posed less risk.

There were many reasons for this state of affairs. In part, our slowness in adapting to a changing COVID-19 landscape was due to the stickiness of our thinking about health conditions. Once we develop an understanding of a particular condition, it is difficult to rethink it. Once we are afraid, it is difficult to accept that the factors that made us afraid to begin with have changed, and we should therefore change our level of fear. A media narrative around COVID-19 that used catchy devices such as case maps and trend arrows and continued to reinforce caseness as the key marker of interest contributed to this mindset. The same was true of how our medical approach influenced our thinking. Hospitalizations, for example, reflected not only disease severity but also availability of hospital beds, meaning that hospitalization for COVID-19 likely evolved over time, as clinicians took advantage of more space to hospitalize those with less severe disease.

In April 2020, shaken by the arrival of a new virus, with an enormous scientific challenge laying ahead, we wanted some clarity about what the COVID-19 endgame might look like. As we went along, it was unclear whether our goalpost should have been fewer cases, fewer severe cases and hospitalizations, or fewer deaths. Or perhaps it should have been all of the above? Meanwhile, our ability to treat and prevent the virus steadily improved. In this way, the public conversation consistently lagged behind our clinical progress in addressing the virus. It turns out we were better at handling COVID-19 than we were at thinking through what we wished to do about COVID-19.

The lesson to take from this is that it benefits us as a society to have clarity about the goalposts for addressing any health challenge. Such clarity comes from a common understanding of what we are trying to achieve. This can point the way to a more effective handling of any crisis, allowing us to focus more intentionally on getting to the goalposts we set and also on reducing collateral harm from poorly informed efforts at prevention as our treatment and containment approaches improve over time.

20

THE LIMITS OF
OUR SCIENCE

The COVID-19 pandemic was characterized in the public space by fractures, mirroring societal divisions and the pitting of science against ideology. This was immensely complicated by President Trump's assumption of strong positions—for example, on the purported utility of hydroxychloroquine as a treatment for COVID-19—that had no basis in scientific fact. Such highly visible support for ideas that were simply wrong, at a time when the world needed clarity without false hope, pushed science to the fore to an unprecedented degree. "Follow the science" became a rallying cry and was part of then presidential candidate Joe Biden's appeal to voters. He promised that he would take the still-evolving COVID-19 science seriously if elected president, in stark contrast to the then incumbent.

Few would argue that science should not be at the heart of decision-making during a pandemic. There is, however, and appropriately, a growing body of work that discusses what science can and cannot do. As we look to learn from the pandemic, it seems worth asking, What are the conditions under which we should be suitably cautious about the science? Three principal conditions come to mind.

The Turning Point. Michael D. Stein and Sandro Galea, Oxford University Press.
© Oxford University Press 2024. DOI: 10.1093/oso/9780197749685.003.0020

First, we should be cautious about science informing decisions about particularly complex systems. Science can indeed shape our understanding of aspects of these systems, yet these narrow aspects are only part of a larger and more intertwined whole. This was perhaps most clearly reflected during the pandemic when it came to decisions about keeping kindergarten through grade 12 schools open. Fairly early on, the science showed that children were at low risk from the virus and did not much influence transmission of COVID-19 in the general population. However, the issue of school opening went beyond a single scientific question. Certainly, there were inputs related to the estimated risks of viral transmission, but there were also risk *perceptions* and issues around the protection of teachers that transcended ready scientific solutions. Scientific engagement on issues that involve different groups with diverse interests need to be focused on particular questions (e.g., How much do children transmit the virus?) but also embedded in larger and more complex societal decision-making.

Second, it is important to remember that scientists bring to their work particular biases, which should lead us to have caution in engaging with scientific pronouncements. There were, for example, perspectives that colored scientists' thinking that were particularly germane to the COVID-19 moment. Notably, academics in universities are increasingly politically left-leaning, and it would not be a stretch to think they might bring this bias to their interpretation of data. This perspective is difficult for scientists to look beyond, particularly when a right-leaning president is sneering at scientific norms and findings. In addition, many of us with post-graduate degrees had the privilege of doing socially and materially better during the pandemic than many other sectors of society, adding a perspective that inevitably informed our work.

Would we, for example, have weighed the burdens of mobility restrictions differently had we been unable to do our jobs with such restrictions in place?

Third, scientists are human, and their approach to the COVID-19 moment was informed by the status that the moment afforded them. We should take such context into account in processing what scientists say. During a high watermark moment for scientific visibility and prestige, it is necessary to marshal the wisdom to recognize the complex and difficult path from science to truth and to beware of overconfidence. Unfortunately, we did not always do so during the pandemic. With future pandemics could well come future boosts in status for science and public health. Learning the lessons of COVID-19 means embracing the humility that lets us navigate such moments with minimal clouding of our judgment.

21

THE NATIONAL CHARACTER

We generally consider a disease a pandemic when it affects multiple countries. By that measure, COVID-19 was a pandemic nearly from the moment it emerged, as the new infection hopscotched from China to Thailand to Japan to South Korea and then to the United States within the span of a month. Just as rapidly as we saw COVID-19 diagnosed in country after country, we began to see dramatically different approaches to containing the disease.

China, for example, adopted a zero-COVID approach that continued throughout most of the pandemic. There, authorities shut down whole neighborhoods and even cities where COVID-19 was detected in an effort to eliminate the virus within its borders. This approach reached draconian extremes, resulting in protests and an eventual lifting of many restrictions. South Korea was an exemplar of a fundamental public health approach to COVID-19, with a national testing effort, contact tracing, and quarantine programs. By contrast, the United States was hit by COVID-19 in the run-up to a federal election, making our response to the pandemic a highly politicized and very public drama. We faltered in implementing testing and generally lurched toward a COVID-19 response characterized by lockdowns of the economy and public

The Turning Point. Michael D. Stein and Sandro Galea, Oxford University Press.
© Oxford University Press 2024. DOI: 10.1003/oso/9780197749685.003.0021

enterprises in the first months of the pandemic. This was followed by a state-by-state patchwork of approaches that persisted several years later.

It is tempting to read the various national responses to COVID-19 as a Rorschach test of national character, of identity. China's ability to pursue a zero-COVID approach rested on its autocratic government that had the power to constrain civil liberties at a moment's notice. These draconian COVID-19 control efforts were an extension of a history of large-scale centrally run programs. South Korea is one of several Southeast Asian countries whose strong bureaucracies support well-funded national programs—informed in no small part by lessons learned during the Middle East Respiratory Syndrome outbreak—which served these countries well in the face of a new viral foe. The American confusion of federal versus state responsibility for COVID-19 mirrored the country's fractured political landscape and long-standing under-investment in public health.

These three countries differed most notably in their chosen measures addressing social practices. China almost completely shut its borders; few Chinese were able to leave the country as the government halted the issuance or renewal of passports. In South Korea, public health sovereignty and expertise were uncontested and policy mandates, such as social distancing and mask-wearing, were adhered to. In the United States, policy fell victim to politics, and often chaos ensued.

In our modern era, we are largely committed to the notion that we have much more in common than we have differences. But it is also clear that history and the dominant cultural conversation about approaches to health were instrumental in shaping the various national responses to COVID-19. Success and failure metrics were moving targets during this protracted pandemic and had been distinctly, nationally, defined in terms of deaths, economic fallout, and government resources utilized. We are now able to reflect, as a global community, on how well each country performed according to these metrics. What did we do that pointed to success or failure during COVID-19, and what implications does this have for future pandemics? The answer lies with both our actions and the national character that informs them.

22

THE RIGHT TO BEAR NEWS

We all experienced the COVID-19 pandemic in different ways. Many of us had COVID-19 or had relatives or friends who contracted the disease or even died from it. Many more experienced changes to activities that were previously routine, such as shopping or travel. On top of our personal experience of the pandemic, we experienced the COVID-19 moment through the lens of the media. This begs the question: How accurate was that view? What if the media narrative was subject to particular biases, coloring the story we consumed, and, as a consequence, shaping how we acted throughout the pandemic?

COVID-19 was a complicated story, with much about it that was truly alarming, much that was neutral, and much that was cause for hope. Yet the media did not always do a good job of reflecting this complexity, skewing instead toward conveying bad news alone. A study published in 2021 suggested that the U.S. media coverage of the pandemic was substantially more negative in tone and framing than coverage in comparable countries. David Leonhardt wrote about this, suggesting that "[the media's] healthy skepticism can turn into reflexive cynicism, and we end up telling something less than the complete story." This assessment is difficult to argue with, given the U.S. media's behavior during the pandemic,

The Turning Point. Michael D. Stein and Sandro Galea, Oxford University Press.
© Oxford University Press 2024. DOI: 10.1093/oso/9780197749685.003.0022

reflecting a bias that complicated our response to the pandemic in several key ways.

First, the tenor of the media narrative had indeed been consistently alarmist, with media outlets seemingly trying to compete with one another to present the daily news as negatively as possible. Improvements in case or death rates in one region were quickly passed over while our attention was drawn to an outbreak in a new location. This focus on the terrible is in some ways characterological for U.S. media, and it long predates COVID-19. Unfortunately, this tendency was particularly troublesome when we were dealing with a rapidly changing pandemic where the collectively experienced narrative was, in real time, shaping policy decisions at the local and national level. Alarmist reports produced perhaps more pessimism and fear than was necessary to inform prudent policy. In some cases, this alarmism actively harmed health. For instance, a relatively small number of children infected led to the widespread closing of schools, despite the long-term harms of school closures to the children.

Second, the negative media narrative set the pace for how we thought of COVID-19 and its consequences. Daily media reports of COVID-19 case counts, for example, did not change until long after vaccines made the severity of caseness much lower than it was at the start of the pandemic. The constant presentation of COVID-19 cases meant one thing before vaccines and another thing altogether once vaccines were on hand. The context had changed (fewer deaths), yet reporting on the top-level case numbers—ubiquitous across media sources—failed to reflect this changing reality, freezing our collective understanding of the disease when it should have changed.

Third, the overwhelming reporting on the negative consequences of COVID-19 came at the expense of reporting on many other challenges to health that were exacerbated by efforts to mitigate the pandemic. For example, there was scant reporting on the dramatic increase in overdose deaths or on mental illness during COVID-19, both of which were linked to limitations on mobility imposed by lockdowns. How may we have considered COVID-19-related lockdowns differently had we seen, for example, daily overdose death numbers reported on the front page of newspapers with the same regularity that we saw daily COVID-19 case counts?

Challenging the general media approach to COVID-19 does not negate the excellent reporting in many media outlets about the pandemic. It should, however, occasion a pause and self-reflection among the media. The media should be proud of its role as arbiter and shaper of the national conversation. But that role comes with responsibility to ensure that negativity bias does not overly influence a story. It is difficult to say that media reporting during COVID-19 fully lived up to that responsibility.

23

THE STORY OF COVID-19

This book is predicated on the idea that COVID-19 represented a turning point in our thinking about the world—and about health. Given that COVID-19 was a pandemic without precedent in our century, that premise seems reasonable enough. But in all the noise generated around COVID-19, what should we remember about the moment? What are the key stories of that time?

First, there is the story of science. The COVID-19 moment represented a triumph of biomedical science. The speed with which a COVID-19 vaccine was developed, supported by mRNA technology, reflected a new era in cutting-edge scientific research. It was an era built on more than a decade of investment in new technology, and one that portended quicker success in vaccination against as-yet-unknown pathogens. It is difficult to envision a future in which we do not see a doubling down on investment in biomedical approaches that can detect novel outbreaks—and develop vaccines to mitigate them—faster, and that seems like a worthwhile societal investment.

Second, there is the story of institutional failures. From political mishandling of the pandemic at the national level, to the use of the pandemic to advance partisan goals, to the politicization of vaccines that led to suboptimal acceptance of this lifesaving

The Turning Point. Michael D. Stein and Sandro Galea, Oxford University Press.
© Oxford University Press 2024. DOI: 10.1093/oso/9780197749685.003.0023

measure (partially negating our biomedical triumph), to the stumbling effort by the national media to convey a clear and dispassionate story about the pandemic, and our public health systems not being adequately prepared to deal with the demands of the moment, our institutions failed us at multiple levels. That is not for a moment to suggest that good people in many places did not do heroic work, but it does call for an honest examination of why our institutions failed and how we can do better.

Third, perhaps the most important story of the COVID-19 moment was the view it afforded of the foundational shortcomings in our social and economic structures. Central to these shortcomings were racial and socioeconomic inequities, stemming from centuries of structural disadvantage, that shape all aspects of how we live, work, and play, and inevitably our health. For example, Black Americans had substantially higher risk of COVID-19 transmission early in the pandemic because they disproportionately worked essential jobs where a shift to remote work was not possible. Similarly, Black Americans were at greater risk of severe COVID-19, due to disproportionate underlying morbidity, stemming from lifetimes of structural racism and disadvantage. None of this was new, but it was brought into plain sight by COVID-19.

As terrible as COVID-19 was for the world, a future outbreak could be just as bad or worse. A future pandemic could combine the high transmissibility of COVID-19 with the far greater lethality of SARS. The better we understand the story of COVID-19, the more it can help inform our efforts to build a world that is less vulnerable to contagion.

24

WHY DID WE CLOSE SCHOOLS?

By March 2020, the COVID-19 pandemic had taken hold in America, and the country had transitioned to an unprecedented slowdown of civic and professional life in an effort to limit the spread of the virus. As part of this general shutdown, kindergarten through grade 12 schools were closed. In spring 2020, 48 states required or recommended the closure of public schools; more than 50 million children and their teachers stayed home. In the face of a new, poorly understood virus, our collective shutdown was entirely reasonable, and to a large extent it was remarkably successful.

And yet, by the summer of 2020, data emerged showing that children were less likely to contract COVID-19, and if they did contract it, their case would likely be mild, and they had a low probability of transmitting it. Data quickly accumulated showing that children were unlikely to be an important source of viral transmission. This, coupled with other data showing the educational and social developmental losses that were being incurred due to persistent school closure—losses often disproportionately affecting marginalized children—made a strong argument for reopening schools in the fall of 2020.

The Turning Point. Michael D. Stein and Sandro Galea, Oxford University Press.
© Oxford University Press 2024. DOI: 10.1093/oso/9780197749685.003.0024

And yet, schools continued to remain closed, affecting as many as half of all children in the United States in the fall of 2020, with only approximately a quarter of schools remaining fully open for in-person learning. Why did schools stay closed when we knew that the risk of them staying closed probably outweighed the risk of them reopening? Likely, there were three key reasons, from which we would do well to learn.

First, the pandemic highlighted the precarious nature of the country's educational infrastructure. On close examination, schools were shown to have poor ventilation and were ill-equipped to implement systemic approaches to testing and screening that would have been required to offer peace of mind to parents and teachers. If a school-based COVID-19 outbreak occurred, could it have been expeditiously contained? The fact that we found ourselves asking that question reflects how we fell short of making schools as safe as they could be.

Second, the politics of school board governance, driven by our particular mix of fear about the unknown virus and lack of confidence that we knew how best to contain the pandemic, paralyzed many school boards from taking quick, decisive action, even when the evidence suggested a way forward. Private schools—often independent, smaller, and better able to mobilize the necessary funding—were able to implement COVID-19 testing and control measures and reopen, whereas public school districts found themselves mired in debate and unable to act swiftly enough to reopen by the fall.

Third, it was never clear if we even saw the need to educate children in-person as a significant priority. This meant that we were not focused enough, nor motivated enough, to invest quickly in the resources needed to overcome the political logjam and enable children to return to school.

This all suggests the need to invest in infrastructure before a crisis; to build effective governance that can plan and act when necessary; and to be clear about what we prioritize, placing the well-being of children, always, above other considerations.

25

THE LIMITS
OF OUR TOLERANCE

In 2021, the Centers for Disease Control and Prevention (CDC) issued new Interim Public Health Recommendations for Vaccinated People, essentially giving a green light to fully vaccinated people to resume activities without wearing a mask or physically distancing. This guidance came just a few weeks after the CDC director noted that she had a sense of "impending doom" as she was watching the pandemic unfold. As such, the guidance, understandably, surprised nearly everyone. It reflected a dramatic pivot point in America's handling of the pandemic, an implicit shift away from community responsibility for COVID-19 transmission toward a more individualistic approach.

Leaving aside arguments over whether this was the correct move based on the science, it was clearly an expression of the CDC's appraisal of what regulation the country could—and could not—bear and an acknowledgment that after a year of COVID-19 restrictions, the country was at the end of its pandemic tolerance.

COVID-19 tested us all. The sum total of pandemic-era experiences set the stage for what we were willing to do to mitigate the spread of the virus.

The Turning Point. Michael D. Stein and Sandro Galea, Oxford University Press.
© Oxford University Press 2024. DOI: 10.1093/oso/9780197749685.003.0025

Any population-wide effort to control disease, whether we acknowledge it explicitly or not, requires the willingness of populations to acquiesce to new rules and regulations, whether these are enforced by the power of law or by emergent social norms. We saw this, to varying degrees, throughout the world during the pandemic. Some countries took a lighter touch to applying pandemic restrictions, whereas others, such as China, tested what populations would tolerate, revealing perhaps the outer limits of the public's willingness to accept restrictions in the name of safety. The pushback faced by approaches perceived as more draconian reflects the importance of public buy-in with regard to the implementation of public health measures.

This buy-in is arguably the decisive factor in determining whether public health recommendations can actually change behavior. For example, rules against smoking indoors only become changes in smoking patterns if, indeed, people choose to comply with them. Similarly, we wear seat belts because of a combination of laws that mandate it and social norms that make seat belt non-use unacceptable. Although we may back up these rules with legal incentives and disincentives, the abject failure of prohibition against alcohol use in the United States a century ago showed that changing the law is not enough to change behavior. Establishing rules of behavior that influence the public's health also requires the consent of populations, and there are limits to the public's tolerance of these rules.

The need for general public agreement had implications during COVID-19. Despite high-profile political arguments about mask-wearing, the public was surprisingly tolerant of policies that encouraged us all to stay home, to not travel, and to limit our interactions for many months. Data showed that most reduced mobility among the population was voluntary, preceding the implementation of regulations that mandated shutdown of businesses and public services, reflecting a general consensus that limitation of movement was, at the time, a good idea. Then, in 2021, the limits of our tolerance began to show. As vaccines became widely available in the spring of 2021, one could sense—and indeed see—the slow dissolution of the public's embrace of lockdowns and masking. Many states dropped post-vaccine guidance, leading to the CDC's change in its recommendations.

We have learned that the public's tolerance for restrictions and actions to promote our collective health is not infinite. This puts pressure, appropriately perhaps, on those who are making the rules to use the best available evidence, but to do so in a way that takes into account what the public may find tolerable over prolonged periods. We should avoid unnecessary rules and focus on ones that are essential, so as not to try the public's patience. Because in cases such as pandemics, our collective tolerance of the rules of engagement is literally a matter of life and death.

26

MISMANAGING MESSAGES

There was never going to be flawless public communication around COVID-19, a new illness that raised an array of novel scientific and sociological issues. Even when we accept this, it is difficult to deny that communication about the pandemic was particularly fraught. The Trump presidency was characterized by repeated lies, and the Biden presidency, at its start, was characterized by perhaps premature optimism and boosterism. Initially looking to a "freedom summer" when we were to be largely over COVID-19, 2021 saw the delta wave sweep the nation and, in the fall of that year, premature scientific statements about the effectiveness of booster vaccines.

In August 2021, President Biden announced that a COVID-19 vaccine booster should be administered to all Americans already vaccinated. "Just remember as a simple rule, eight months after your second shot, get a booster shot," Biden said, promising a booster rollout in a month. Federal health agencies then weighed in, and their opinions had to be shoehorned into the basic shape Biden had offered so as not to contradict his original statement. Yet a month later, when the vaccine was to be available "to all," only one type of booster had been approved, and only for the elderly, persons with workplace exposure to COVID-19, nursing home

The Turning Point. Michael D. Stein and Sandro Galea, Oxford University Press.
© Oxford University Press 2024. DOI: 10.1003/oso/9780197749685.003.0026

residents, and immunocompromised people who had received that type of vaccine originally.

The confusion about whether boosters should be taken, and by whom, reflected what happens when policymakers jump to too-simple conclusions based on still-unsettled science. When Biden made his announcement, no one really knew the connection between antibody responses (which the booster promised to increase) and duration of human protection. Whether boosters would actually protect against infection, or reinfection, was simply not clear. This, then, complicated our thinking around boosters, raising the question of why we needed boosters to begin with. Was the aim of a booster to reduce ongoing viral spread by curbing, at least temporarily, milder infections? This could seem redundant because the initial vaccinations were continuing to limit the worst effects of COVID-19 in the United States. Would a booster, urgently delivered, save lives? And should we really have been focusing on additional vaccinations for Americans before the elderly and health workers in many low-income countries could receive a single dose?

Eventually, we saw the staggered approval and release of the Pfizer and Moderna boosters, which, along with different timing of booster administration and sizing of doses, made messaging around them difficult. The mix-and-match strategy that allowed physicians to administer a different COVID-19 vaccine as a booster than the one patients had initially received was a boon to vaccine recipients but also involved its own confusion. Some health care providers and pharmacies even needed charts to help them keep things straight. Meanwhile, the very need for boosters gave the ever-eager anti-vaxxers new ammunition to say that vaccines were not working. The message around the implementation and rollout of original vaccines in December 2020 was far simpler: Vaccination will save lives. Still, much of the American public remained unvaccinated. It is difficult to see how this proportion would have been much higher for receipt of boosters given the more convoluted messaging around their rollout.

The credibility and consistency of federal messages are foundational to our best public health efforts. State health officials rely on federal precision to promote and support local efforts. Public health requires clear messaging, the admission of uncertainty, and the avoidance of overly pat solutions. Even so, it can be difficult to hit all the right notes.

27

THE VACCINATION GLASS
HALF FULL

The time of polio was a time of shared national fear. This fear helped drive the search for a vaccine and informed public jubilation when a vaccine finally arrived. With 21,000 Americans paralyzed in the year before a vaccine was licensed, doses of the Salk vaccine were being manufactured before the first large clinical trial was complete. This would be echoed by the development and testing of Moderna and Pfizer vaccines in 2020. Yet by 1957, two years after the Salk inoculation was available, only half of the adult population younger than age 40 years had received at least one shot. Even by 1961, only 77 percent had received one dose, 67 percent the full three doses. This reflects a core truth: It has always been difficult to vaccinate Americans. The challenge of vaccinating the population for COVID-19 was no exception.

What accounts for this difficultly? We could blame a number of factors, including mistrust in government and an undermining of authority of all kinds—scientists, judges, intelligence agencies, and corporate leaders. And yet, given our national history of vaccine hesitancy, it should have come as no surprise that there were so many vaccine holdouts in the COVID-19 era. After all, in the years before COVID-19, less than half of eligible adults received an

The Turning Point. Michael D. Stein and Sandro Galea, Oxford University Press.
© Oxford University Press 2024. DOI: 10.1093/oso/9780197749685.003.0027

influenza vaccine, and approximately one-third agreed to hepatitis B vaccination or to a shingles vaccine (for those older than age 60 years).

The polio vaccine's initial target was children, and vaccinators knew exactly where to go to find this population: schools. As a result, school-age children (aged 5–14 years) had the highest levels of polio vaccination; approximately 93 percent had at least one dose, and 87 percent had completed the non-mandated series of three inoculations within the first two years. Unlike polio, COVID-19's vaccine rollout started with adults—the population at higher risk of COVID-19 and its complications. This made the task more difficult. America's 250 million adults were spread all over the country, making it more difficult to vaccinate them efficiently. Public health officials had to find ways to create an infrastructure for rapid vaccination that did not previously exist. To make matters more difficult, COVID-19 vaccination entailed several complicating procedures; for example, people had to wait 15 minutes following vaccination to make sure they did not have an allergic reaction, and there were restrictions on who could receive a vaccine in the early months of 2020, as priority groups went first.

Then there was the factor of simple loss of interest in multiple vaccinations. This was seen in declining rates of booster uptake among the U.S. population—an underdiscussed phenomenon in the context of the vaccine conversation. This decline was notable among older adults, the population most at risk of COVID with, arguably, the most personal stake in keeping their vaccination status current. As of October 2022, only approximately 44 percent of Americans older than age 65 years had received the second booster, compared to 71 percent who received the first.

All of this suggests that the national challenges with vaccinating the population are substantial and neither new nor, when viewed in historical context, surprising. Compounding these challenges, disinformation at a scale and speed previously unseen helped spread irrational fears about vaccine side effects. This sometimes overwhelmed rational fears about a deadly virus and slowed vaccination efforts further. During COVID-19, we were more politically polarized than at any time in recent memory, which informed the partisan gap in COVID-19 vaccinations and deaths.

Polio was a shared national tragedy, but COVID-19 was not seen this way, complicating national efforts toward a coherent, "we are all in this together" approach. Reclaiming a sense of shared collective experience could help shape a more effective vaccination effort in the future.

SECTION 3

ETHICS

HEALTH rests on a foundation of values, ethics. These ethics shape how we invest in health, how we prioritize care in times of crisis, whether we pursue an equitable distribution of the resources that generate health, and more. As we reflect on COVID-19, it is worth examining how unresolved ethical considerations complicated our response to the pandemic and how we can do better in the future.

28

TIME FOR AN ETHICS REFRESH?

Imagine news emerges of a novel coronavirus outbreak in Uganda. Within weeks, it becomes clear that the new virus, previously not found in humans, is spreading rapidly and may have a case fatality rate that is higher than that of COVID-19. The world starts bracing for a new pandemic.

Meanwhile, scientists announce that using the widely available viral sequence, they have created an mRNA vaccine that they believe will be safe and efficacious in humans. They say Phase 1 and Phase 2 safety trials will be completed soon, followed by a large-scale, Phase 3 effectiveness trial, enrolling tens of thousands of volunteers.

Can we expedite this process? Doing so raises an important ethical question: Should we be moving ahead with mass vaccine administration before having completed a Phase 3 trial? Clearly the answer today in most Western democracies would be no, we should not vaccinate prior to completing Phase 3 trials. It has been a tenet of vaccine implementation that we want to ascertain mass safety and effectiveness before we distribute to the wider population.

The Turning Point. Michael D. Stein and Sandro Galea, Oxford University Press.
© Oxford University Press 2024. DOI: 10.1093/oso/9780197749685.003.0018

But in 2020, Russia and China took a different approach. The two countries developed, respectively, the Sputnik V and Sinovac vaccines, and they proceeded with mass vaccination, likely reaching millions of people, well before the end of the vaccines' Phase 3 trials. In the case of China, these efforts were likely helped by the country's zero-COVID policy, which used severe social policing to enforce pandemic policies. The Russian and Chinese vaccines had variable efficacy, although Sputnik V's efficacy and safety were later confirmed to be comparable to vaccines adopted in the West. Notably, the Russian and Chinese efforts to vaccinate their populations before the completion of Phase 3 trials were largely met by skepticism in the Western press and in academic conversations. In China, the test of its vaccine's effectiveness began in earnest when the government lifted its zero-COVID policy, opening the country to a surge of cases.

Might our view, in the West, of the ethics of expedited vaccine distribution change? Certainly, our ethical norms about when we should deploy biological solutions to novel viral assaults have changed before. During the AIDS epidemic, in no small part due to ACT UP activism, what we considered to be ethical in the context of regulatory approval was rethought, and we established pathways for much faster delivery of lifesaving drugs that were being held up by our pre-AIDS standards.

Is it time for new, post-COVID-19 ethical standards for how we approve and deploy vaccines? Perhaps. It seems to us that there is much to learn from the COVID-19 vaccine rollout and that it is reasonable to ask, How many lives could we have saved, how much faster could we have restarted our economy, had we started mass vaccination as China did in July instead of December 2020 (taking care, of course, to create a context of informed consent that was honest about what we did and did not know at that time about the vaccine's effects)? It is important to consider this question now, to develop a clear sense of what we will and will not accept in this area. The time to think carefully about our ethics is before, not during, the next pandemic.

29

WHO GOES FIRST?

To return to the example of the Salk polio vaccine, it is worth noting that the rollout did not go smoothly for reasons other than just vaccine hesitancy. In April 1955, the vaccination effort was characterized by critical shortages. When the vaccine was approved, the Secretary of Health, Education, and Welfare did not have a single injection available. Funding was also an issue—the campaign to cure polio was to be funded by charitable donations. But the polio vaccine rollout did have one key element in its favor: There was a clear priority system—a waiting line with the youngest and most vulnerable kids first.

The situation was different with the rollout of the COVID-19 vaccine. The epidemiology of the disease was such that children were not a priority. So, who was? Although most states had the elderly and health care workers at the front of the line, followed by those with severe health risks, it was not at all clear how we should have prioritized within each group. Should people of color have been offered priority spots, given the greater risk they faced? Were risks additive? Should we have prioritized vaccination in geographic hot spots?

Our confusion in addressing these questions stemmed, in part, from the complex epidemiology of COVID-19 itself. But it also

The Turning Point. Michael D. Stein and Sandro Galea, Oxford University Press.
© Oxford University Press 2024. DOI: 10.1093/oso/9780197749685.003.0029

came from the fact that we had not developed a shared comprehensive economic or moral theory for weighting our different goals. Is a younger life worth more than an elderly life because the younger person presumably has more life left? Should groups who act irresponsibly (those, for example, who refused to wear masks during COVID-19) paradoxically receive the benefit of a vaccine early to protect others, or should they be left with a longer wait?

Absent an agreed upon vocabulary of risk weighting, we are driven, then, to politics. This is perhaps not surprising. Public health always intersects with the work of distributing the resources and socioeconomic capital that support health—which is to say, the work of politics. But the balance between public health and politics in the COVID-19 moment was so skewed toward politics that it often made public health considerations come in a distant second. Elected state officials prioritized vaccine distribution based on local political exigency. In Colorado, for example, ski industry employees living in congregate settings were part of the early vaccine rounds. Representatives in Georgia and Arkansas included workers in meatpacking and food processing plants.

It surely is one of the central lessons of the COVID-19 moment that we need to invest in doing the difficult work of deciding how to prioritize rare and important supplies before, not during, a crisis. Absent that, we are left with little more than special interests jockeying to determine which lives are saved first. This should be unacceptable to us.

30

WHAT'S MOST IMPORTANT?

The degree of protection afforded by any vaccine can be understood in terms of its efficacy or effectiveness. The distinction between the two terms is important. *Efficacy* refers to the reduction in biologically proven illness (detected serologically or via culture of the virus from the patient), whereas *effectiveness* refers to the reduction in clinical consequences, which for infectious disease such as influenza or COVID-19 include pneumonia, hospitalization, and death.

The influenza vaccine has a variable efficacy; it is not terrific at preventing infections (functioning at 50 percent efficacy) in years during which the vaccine is not well matched to circulating strains of the virus. But it performs much better (functioning at 90 percent efficacy) when it is well matched. However, the more important purpose of getting vaccinated is preventing hospitalizations and deaths. On this score, the flu vaccine reduces hospitalization by 90 percent in healthy adults. More important, it decreases the risk of death in the elderly, in whom most deaths occur, by 20–50 percent.

The story of COVID-19 and its vaccines was in some ways unhelpfully influenced by our confusion about efficacy and

The Turning Point. Michael D. Stein and Sandro Galea, Oxford University Press.
© Oxford University Press 2024. DOI: 10.1093/oso/9780197749685.003.0030

effectiveness. Media reports had focused far too much on overall efficacy, which fundamentally was concerned with limiting the risk of acquiring the virus, as marked by counts of "cases" (i.e., persons who tested positive). However, for a virus for which a substantial proportion of cases were asymptomatic, and with a majority of cases presenting mild respiratory symptoms, a key measure of interest should have been less viral spread than the number of severe cases. Clearly, limiting spread also mattered, primarily in order to limit the risk to those who were susceptible to severe disease. Our focus on "flattening the curve" was an effort to ensure that fewer people were sick at any one time, to make sure that the health care system could cope with severe cases of the virus. The burden on health systems—the need to ration intensive care beds and ventilators—is appreciably different depending on the severity of the illness.

However, based on our experience with influenza, the key measure in our COVID-19 vaccine discussion should have been observations about limiting severe disease and death. Unfortunately, the media conversation around the 2021 announcement of the Johnson & Johnson vaccine release was dominated almost exclusively by the vaccine's overall 66 percent efficacy, while largely failing to note that the vaccine was 85 percent effective against severe disease. And the conversation about the Johnson & Johnson vaccine was broadly reflective of our muddled conversation about the efficacy and effectiveness of vaccines in general during COVID-19. Core to our thinking during the crisis should have been avoiding severity of disease and death. This was particularly true as the disease evolved and confronted us with new variants, and the biology of the disease became clearer with the revelation that we could be infected time and again and that booster vaccines would still be beneficial. Instead, we lost our focus on the fundamentals—the power of vaccines to prevent severe disease and death—to the detriment of the vaccine conversation.

31

ACHIEVING HEALTH EQUITY, EFFICIENTLY

Public health has long faced challenges in balancing the sometimes-competing demands of equity and efficiency. *Health equity*, one of the core principles that animates public health, suggests that we should implement any health-related effort such that those who are most vulnerable are protected first. *Efficiency* refers to the success of our efforts in promoting the overall health of populations. Much, if not most, of the time, these goals are aligned. We can promote population health while leading, first, with promoting the health of those who are most vulnerable. And when the two principles are in conflict, it is probably right, most of the time, to privilege health equity, to help push against the injustice that has left some groups lagging on health.

With that in mind, it is worth applauding the principles that informed the rollout of the COVID-19 vaccine in the United States. Although prior chapters of this book have been critical of aspects of the rollout, there was indeed much to praise. Broadly speaking, guidelines prioritized vaccination of health care providers and persons at high risk of contracting COVID-19, ensuring that these groups were vaccinated before others. This approach correctly recognized that those at higher risk needed to be protected first,

The Turning Point. Michael D. Stein and Sandro Galea, Oxford University Press.
© Oxford University Press 2024. DOI: 10.1093/oso/9780197749685.003.0031

and most states embraced these principles and implemented their vaccination plans accordingly, even establishing fines for any vaccine providers who did not comply with these guidelines.

This was where the rubber met the road during the vaccination process, and it was where we saw conflicts between equity and efficiency. As states moved forward with implementing equitable vaccine distribution plans, large swaths of the population were told that they would not be eligible to receive the vaccine for months, as equity considerations led to certain groups being placed at the front of the line. Stories quickly emerged of challenges with this system. In several jurisdictions, there was evidence that some vaccines were being wasted, with persons at high risk not yet allowed to receive them. Distribution centers were being underused, informal systems of vaccine distribution emerged, and states quickly tried to amend rules to expand risk tiers to deal with these logistical challenges.

This brought us to an interesting juncture in the COVID-19 moment. Efforts to be equitable with vaccine distribution clearly introduced inefficiencies into the system, and we witnessed public displeasure with the slow rate of vaccine distribution. What should we have learned from this moment? We perhaps should have seen that efforts to ensure equity may be viewed, in the public narrative, as the reason for inefficiencies. This reinforces the importance of communicating why equity should be at the heart of decision-making, by conveying to the public the challenge of disproportionately borne risk and the collective responsibility we have to rectify inequities, even if this comes at the cost of some inefficiencies.

32

THE LONG SHADOW
OF MEDICAL RACISM

In the first decades of the 20th century, medical experts insisted that the Black population was not susceptible to polio, based on presumed biological differences between Black people and White people that had, conversely, also been used to allege that Blacks were more vulnerable to syphilis.

There is, of course, no racial difference in susceptibility to polio, or to syphilis, or to most other medical conditions. There *are* substantial racial differences in how we treat medical conditions, and an equally long history of grappling with whether to support a more equitable approach to treating these conditions.

This is well illustrated by a historical anecdote. President Franklin Roosevelt claimed he had overcome polio at Warm Springs polio rehabilitation center. During the 1936 presidential campaign, Roosevelt was confronted about the center's all-White admission policy. Roosevelt, who enjoyed extraordinary support among Black voters, responded by announcing, in 1937, the formation of the National Foundation for Infantile Paralysis (later called the March of Dimes), which soon became the nation's largest disease philanthropy and quickly announced "the disease attacked all races."

The Turning Point. Michael D. Stein and Sandro Galea, Oxford University Press.
© Oxford University Press 2024. DOI: 10.1093/oso/9780197749685.003.0032

The March of Dimes went on to play an outsize role in the eventual trials of the polio vaccine. In the massive clinical trial of the Salk polio vaccine, begun in 1954 and funded by the March of Dimes, Black children were included, enrolled at the Tuskegee Infantile Paralysis Center. It was the year of the *Brown v. Board of Education* ruling, and the integration of Black and White professionals made news as White nurses assisted Black physicians in administering the vaccine to Black children. The new science of polio, however, did not counter the pervasive medical racism of the time—Warm Springs remained segregated, separate hospitals and treatment persisted, and White children got preference over Black children when the Salk vaccine administration rollout began in 1955.

We have now been through another moment when public health, politics, and civil rights activism converged. COVID-19 exposed racial inequities in access to and quality of medical care. The country's latest mass inoculation program provided a test of whether we could break the inequities of the current health care and public health systems and whether new trust could be fostered among vaccine recipients. This vaccination program was dependent on Americans believing that the initial, limited supplies of doses would be allocated fairly—to those who needed them most, rather than to those with the most political clout or historic advantage. Clearly, this trust was not fully present, particularly among communities of color. That we have fallen short of addressing racial bias in how we prevent and treat disease may partially account for this, and reflect the importance of doing better in the future.

33

HEALTH INEQUITIES
BEYOND COVID-19

In 2020, COVID-19 was the third leading cause of death in the United States for persons older than age 45 years, and it was the second leading cause of death for persons older than age 85 years. Clearly, the virus represented a cataclysmic event for health. Yet it is important to see the catastrophe of the pandemic in a broader perspective—as difficult as this can be.

In any given year, almost 3 million Americans die—the leading causes of death being heart disease, with approximately 650,000 annual deaths, and cancer, with approximately 600,000 annual deaths. These deaths reflect a range of health inequities, many of which came to the fore during the pandemic. It is now important to apply what we learned about these inequities during the pandemic to improving U.S. health going forward.

The disproportionate burden of COVID-19 borne by people of color was perhaps the most glaring of the health inequities we saw during the pandemic. It reflected the unfairness that underlies health inequities, motivating us to address systematic forces such as structural racism as a means of tackling these inequities.

But socioeconomic forces such as racism are relevant not just in the context of COVID-19. The deep and entrenched socioeconomic

The Turning Point. Michael D. Stein and Sandro Galea, Oxford University Press.
© Oxford University Press 2024. DOI: 10.1093/oso/9780197749685.003.0033

inequities that drove COVID-19 influence nearly *all* other deaths in the United States. In an analysis, sociologist Elizabeth Wrigley-Field estimated that 400,000 excess White deaths would be needed to raise White mortality to the best-ever Black mortality; it would take 700,000 excess White deaths to narrow the Black–White life expectancy gap. This analysis suggests that the scope of death from COVID-19 is comparable to the scope of the Black–White mortality gap in general, *every year*.

As we study the health gaps exposed by COVID-19, it seems important not to lose sight of what now has become apparent to all—that the health gaps that existed long before COVID-19 will continue to exist without clear-eyed and focused action. Can we now think creatively about ways to bridge seemingly intractable racial and socioeconomic health gaps? Can we use this point in time to argue for foundational investments in, for example, efforts that can close racial wealth gaps, universal access to health care, or wholesale investment in affordable housing that leaves no group behind? Some of these ideas may have been politically untenable before COVID-19. We should not let the opportunity we now have to advance them pass.

34

A HARD WEIGHT

Long before COVID-19, obesity was a serious health concern, a major contributor to cardiovascular and cancer deaths. More than one in three adults in the United States are living with obesity, and many more are overweight. The arrival of COVID-19 shed new light on this long-standing health problem. The pandemic led many Americans—housebound, exercising less, drinking more alcohol, depressed—to gain weight.

At the same time, it became clear that being overweight worsened COVID-19 outcomes. Obesity tripled the risk of hospitalization and increased intensive care unit admission and death from COVID-19, particularly for those younger than age 65 years in the United States. Internationally, nearly 90 percent of deaths from the pandemic had been in countries with high levels of obesity. Only old age was a stronger risk factor of severe illness.

The interconnectedness of certain health conditions is unfortunately clearest when viewed through the lens of race. In the United States, non-Hispanic Black adults have the highest prevalence of self-reported obesity (39.8 percent), followed by Hispanic adults, with non-Hispanic White adults reporting rates 10 percent lower. Part of the reason that Hispanic and

The Turning Point. Michael D. Stein and Sandro Galea, Oxford University Press.
© Oxford University Press 2024. DOI: 10.1093/oso/9780197749685.003.0034

non-Hispanic Black adults suffered worse outcomes from COVID-19 is obesity. And much of the obesity story is a poverty story: Unhealthy foods are simply more available and affordable. Persistent food insecurity due to decreased affordability, particularly among those with low incomes or who are out of work, leads to a diet of cheap and energy-dense foods and sugar-loaded drinks.

Of course, the causes and trajectories of obesity are complex. Neighborhood design matters. Campaigns for healthier eating matter. Food policies that work at scale in schools as well as supermarkets matter. And, of course, personal responsibility matters. To make societal headway, environmental and economic policies need to meet up with the psychology of food preferences; incentives for sellers and shoppers need to align with advertising and labeling edicts. And cultural norms around eating should be encouraged to align with healthier choices.

Our long record of societal pressures that induce many to gain weight, and the increased risk of severe COVID-19 that this caused, should be a lesson. Fewer overweight Americans would have reduced the number of emergency room visits and hospitalizations during the pandemic, just as fewer overweight Americans would mean a healthier country now.

Making sustained progress means addressing the structural drivers of obesity. The power of the food and beverage industry is overwhelming and difficult to oppose, with meaningful change dependent on politically problematic words: taxes and bans. Yet modest taxes on sugary drinks produce only modest effects. Unhealthy foods are simply cheaper—making them less so is key to discouraging their consumption.

It is worth remembering that respiratory viruses *before* COVID-19 produced worse consequences in persons living with excess body weight. This means we are primed to fail during the next pandemic if we do not address the challenge of obesity. We should do so, while we still have time.

35

MANDATING VACCINES

The triumph amid the tragedy of the COVID-19 moment was the rapid development of safe, effective vaccines. Vaccines are costly and slow to develop, and yet we had two, from Pfizer–BioNTech and Moderna, available within approximately eight months of the arrival of COVID-19 in the United States, each with more than 90 percent effectiveness. That was a remarkable technical achievement and represents the culmination of years of investment in the development of mRNA as a viable vaccine delivery platform. The rollout of vaccines at the beginning of 2021 was met with understandable enthusiasm and predictions of a "summer of freedom" when, the thinking went, sufficient numbers of people would be vaccinated to essentially curtail the spread of the COVID-19 pandemic.

And yet, once vaccines were made widely available, uptake was far slower than had been generally anticipated. Although a substantial proportion of Americans rushed to get vaccines, the number of people willing to get vaccinated soon stalled, with more than one-third of Americans hesitating or downright refusing. This, reasonably enough, occasioned its fair share of public consternation and discussion about how best to increase the proportion of vaccinated Americans.

The Turning Point. Michael D. Stein and Sandro Galea, Oxford University Press.
© Oxford University Press 2024. DOI: 10.1093/oso/9780197749685.003.0035

This conversation, perhaps inevitably, turned to mandating vaccines for adults, recognizing that this could create the conditions for a more rapid return to "normal" functioning. Many workplaces did indeed mandate vaccination. This was initially a phenomenon of private workplaces, but it soon extended to public sector employers such as fire departments and school systems. The question then extended—again, perhaps inevitably—to whether we could, or should, mandate vaccines for all adults.

This book will leave to others a discussion about the ethics of vaccine mandates for adults—it is indeed a subject for longer consideration. However, it is worth noting here some pragmatic concerns raised by the issue of vaccine mandates.

First, the mechanics of widespread vaccine mandates for all adults are daunting and next to impossible in a pluralist society. Operationally, how would we have identified defiant adults? What would we have done once we did? Would we have penalized or arrested them? Such difficult questions are unavoidable when considering how mandates would work in practice.

Second, stripping access to public services from the unvaccinated can quickly lead to restricting access to fundamental rights of citizenship, putting the very idea of a vaccine mandate at odds with what we think citizens can reasonably expect. Would we, for example, have denied the unvaccinated access to post offices, social security offices, and even hospitals?

Third, although the COVID-19 vaccines that were available were extraordinarily safe and effective, the bar for a state-mandated treatment or vaccine of any kind needs to be sufficiently high as to be, without a shadow of a doubt, not only completely safe but also completely necessary.

Fourth, as COVID-19 evolved, as well as our ability to treat it, so did the consequences of catching the disease, with implications for the conversation about vaccine mandates. It is very different to mandate vaccines for a new disease with potentially serious, largely unknown effects and high mortality among older adults than it is to mandate vaccines for a disease we know much about and can effectively treat. However, even under the most urgent conditions, mandates are not to be adopted lightly, and it is right that we should have a robust, data-informed conversation about their costs and benefits.

Fundamentally, in applying a universal vaccine mandate, we would need to weigh whether the cost would be justified, particularly given the amount of resistance and antagonism a mandate could generate among the public. All in all, we should fall on the side of extreme caution when it comes to considering efforts such as a population-wide vaccine mandate.

36

LEAVING
THE WORLD BEHIND

About a year into the widespread availability of vaccines, more than 220 million Americans, two-thirds of the population, received at least one dose of the COVID-19 vaccine. Meanwhile, approximately half of the world's population had received at least one dose, even as only 3.7 percent of people in low-income countries received one. This glaring vaccine inequity raises discomfiting questions. What is the responsibility of the high-income world to the health of the low-income world? What can we do better to level the global playing field with regard to health?

Discrepancies in vaccination are, of course, not new. They reflect a global status quo that has long been divided into health haves and have nots. For example, in 2019, life expectancy at birth in Nigeria was approximately 54 years; in Japan, it was 84 years. That we countenance a 30-year gap in life expectancy across countries—that humans have such different life trajectories linked to accident of birth—should trouble us much more than it does. The COVID-19 vaccination gap was simply one further

The Turning Point. Michael D. Stein and Sandro Galea, Oxford University Press.
© Oxford University Press 2024. DOI: 10.1093/oso/9780197749685.003.0036

reminder of dramatic global gaps in health achievement—of how far we have to go to get to global health equity.

Grappling with this challenge means first grappling with a foundational question: Why do we have health gaps to begin with? The answer emerges from an understanding of what causes health. Health is, at core, a product of the conditions of living—factors such as the availability of clean air, drinkable water, safe food, opportunities for stable housing, safe transportation, and a livable wage. The gap in health achievement across countries mirrors a gap in the availability of salutary assets for people in different countries. Therefore, narrowing health gaps requires narrowing asset gaps and rectifying long-standing global wealth asymmetries. This is, needless to say, a substantial challenge, one that runs counter to much of how the world is currently shaped. The global order rests on a status quo of inequities—global supply chains, for example, are predicated on cheaper costs of labor in low-income countries supplying goods to high-income countries. Is it then realistic to imagine a world in which we shift the global order to the end of promoting health equity?

The enormous gaps in vaccination throughout the world reflect long-standing health gaps, and those health gaps are a reflection of an imbalance in global assets. In this context, COVID-19 was a teachable moment for health. It is now on all of us to learn to identify how we can do better. It is worth remembering that 80 percent of the 5.5 billion vaccinations delivered in the first nine months of vaccine availability occurred in high- and middle-income countries. Having billions of people un- or undervaccinated created reservoirs of SARS-CoV-2 infection that threatened health all around the world; this is a reminder that the world is healthier overall only if all are healthy, not just a few. In the spirit of this being a turning point moment, should not the experience of a pandemic spur us to think critically about how we can move toward global health equity? If not now, when?

37

DIGITAL SURVEILLANCE

COVID-19 was the first pandemic to go viral in both the physical and digital space. The beginning of the pandemic was accompanied by a range of predictions about our coming use of digital technologies to monitor pandemic spread. Early on, exposure notification and contact-tracing apps that were in a position to help keep countries open before a vaccine was available were much discussed. Although at least 24 states and Washington, DC, rolled out exposure notification apps through Google and Apple's Exposure Notification framework, few of these made any perceptible inroads into the broader population management of COVID-19. Other countries were more agile. Singapore, South Korea, and Israel enlisted technology, including mobile apps, to facilitate their contact tracing and pandemic management.

The appeal of digital technology to help control pandemic spread is readily apparent. Traditional contact tracing is labor-intensive, involving phone calls, interviews, footwork, and detailed investigation. Digital technologies can reduce some of that work, supporting greater effectiveness in our response to a pandemic. But if utilized widely and found to be efficacious, one question would immediately arise: Given the intersection of digital

The Turning Point. Michael D. Stein and Sandro Galea, Oxford University Press.
© Oxford University Press 2024. DOI: 10.1093/oso/9780197749685.003.0037

technologies with personal data, could we balance protecting public health with safeguarding civil liberties?

Some of the app deployment in the United States provided early hints about the potentially intrusive aspects of this technology. North and South Dakota's COVID-19 apps were found to have secretly violated users' privacy by sharing location data and personal identifiers with corporate third parties. More than location trackers, a few apps also employed facial recognition and physiological surveillance. In the name of COVID-19 exposure minimization, some American colleges mandated app use to track students' whereabouts to ensure that they never left campus.

The questions raised by infectious disease-related apps are complex and will likely be with us for some time. They include the following: Will a specific app's use be mandatory? Can data be used by authorities other than public health officials, such as law enforcement, where warrantless contact tracing violates the Fourth Amendment? Will an app collect only those data elements needed for public health, and is the policy and design around app use transparent? When are data destroyed and do users get to choose that timing? Then there is the emerging challenge of artificial intelligence (AI). The tensions between civil liberties and the need for rapid public health response are exacerbated with the use of AI in the context of a pandemic. Yet AI is, according to one computer scientist, "the new electricity." It is ubiquitous, embedded in the internet itself, its influence difficult—perhaps impossible—to avoid.

Digital surveillance technologies never became a centerpiece of the public health effort against COVID-19 in the United States. Perhaps this was fortuitous given the number of open questions that remain about the role that such approaches can play in a society that values privacy and autonomy. Yet we cannot dodge these questions forever.

38

BALANCING AUTONOMY AND INDIVIDUAL RESPONSIBILITY

There is a Ghanaian proverb, "You cannot cry harder than the bereaved." The proverb suggests that our capacity to help ease the suffering of others is, sadly, limited. It is a reminder that it behooves us to have the humility to recognize this limitation. During COVID-19, the message of this proverb was useful, as we attempted to navigate the complicated balance of individual autonomy—what we need to do for ourselves—and collective responsibility—what we can do for each other.

The tug of war around the use of face masks was the first and most visible example of our efforts to strike this balance. Although the issue was cynically exploited for political ends, at heart it was a classic push–pull between those who wished for maximum individual autonomy and those who advocated for collective responsibility. A fair, public health–focused look at the issue suggests that the latter readily outweighed the former. Mask-wearing is an inconvenience, but a relatively minor one, and the case that wearing a mask protects others is strong. The kind of trade-off this reflects

The Turning Point. Michael D. Stein and Sandro Galea, Oxford University Press.
© Oxford University Press 2024. DOI: 10.1093/oso/9780197749685.003.0038

is far from unprecedented. We have as a society often decided that we are willing to limit some individual autonomy for a readily apparent public good. For example, worries about the risk of secondhand smoke were critical in the adoption of indoor smoking bans, as we collectively accepted that it was worth limiting the freedom of some to smoke anywhere in order to preserve the freedom of many from unwanted cancer risk. In keeping with this logic, the majority of U.S. states put in place mask mandates or other forms of masking requirements during the pandemic.

But as the pandemic evolved, the balance of individual freedoms and collective responsibilities became more complicated, particularly around the issue of vaccination. Early in the vaccination effort, it was clear that many did not have ready access to vaccines and, as such, we had a collective responsibility to continue preserving limits on our individual freedoms—through measures such as physical distancing, masking, and restricted availability of entertainment venues—until everyone had the opportunity to be vaccinated, to ensure we could all be protected.

But what about when vaccines are genuinely abundantly available during a pandemic and some people still refuse to be vaccinated? The reasons why some make this choice are, of course, complicated, often resting on deeply entrenched, entirely legitimate, historical mistrusts. But at what point during a pandemic, assuming the emergence of a safe and readily available vaccine, can we reasonably expect individuals to get vaccinated so that we can restore society to normal functioning? In other words, when do we say that our collective responsibility has been fulfilled, and now it is on individuals to choose whether or not to protect themselves?

Then there is the question of just who are we vaccinating *for*? The question takes on urgency when, for example, we are discussing the vaccination of young children, a group at lower risk of COVID-19. Are we primarily vaccinating kids for their own health or to protect the adults around them? Likewise, when we mandate masks in schools, are we doing it to protect kids or their teachers? These are difficult, perhaps uncomfortable questions. But they are necessary if we are to learn from the pandemic moment to pursue policies founded on a reasonable cost–benefit analysis. It is neither fair nor in the best interests of health for the health of the few to come at the expense of the well-being of the many.

39

PROFITS AND PROFITEERING

During the COVID-19 pandemic, approximately 40 million Americans filed for unemployment payments. Meanwhile, 40 new billionaires took their places on the world's richest lists, with many new fortunes created by the pandemic. Culture war grifters made new fortunes selling alternatives to vaccines. Foreign swindlers took advantage of the huge transfer of wealth from federal programs to U.S. households. Although the era of the COVID-19 pandemic was about human lives, it also turned out to be a boon for capitalism.

Executives and the biochemists with stakes in the companies that developed vaccines made incredible profits, as did those running the contract research organizations that directed the clinical trials and those directing the glass manufacturing businesses that made vials for the vaccines. Riches came to those who led companies that made gowns and face masks, gloves and hand sanitizers, and to those who produced diagnostic tests, digital X-ray analysis systems, and pulmonary products such as oximeters. Those who created software for scheduling appointments at mass vaccination sites also did well, as did antibody treatment manufacturers and home delivery services.

The Turning Point. Michael D. Stein and Sandro Galea, Oxford University Press.
© Oxford University Press 2024. DOI: 10.1093/oso/9780197749685.003.0039

For a time, the need for vaccines muted objections to the vast profits drug companies stood to make during the pandemic and the role the public purse was playing in underwriting these profits. Vaccines were one area in which the engine of capitalism seemed an unalloyed good, the promise of riches helping supercharge development of something many desperately wanted. However, as boosters began to roll out like so many iPhone updates, the companies making them started to look less like saviors and more like what they are—profit-oriented businesses. This is not to say, of course, that boosters were not needed and did not do much good, or that drug companies did not play a decisive role in making the pandemic more manageable. But as our treatments for COVID-19 got better, and vaccines helped end the most acute phase of the pandemic, conversations about the costs and benefits of regular booster uptake complicated the public's view of vaccines and the companies making them.

At the same time, medical misinformers also found financial opportunity. Fraudsters with large social media followings sold natural health "cures" and vitamin supplements as alternatives to vaccines. America's Frontline Doctors, a group working against vaccinations, convinced tens of thousands of Americans to seek telemedicine consultations, while selling millions of dollars of ineffective medications. The anti-parasitic drug ivermectin, sold online, was promoted as an effective treatment for COVID-19 despite having no proven anti-viral benefits but clear harms when overused. Hydroxychloroquine, an anti-malarial pill, was endorsed by a president and sold by his followers for both preventing and treating COVID-19. Yet meta-analysis had shown that it was useless against COVID-19 and could lead to potentially fatal cardiac complications. These medical misdirections undermined public health messaging while making a tidy profit for those who promoted them.

During the time of pandemic, new markets opened, and profit-driven schemes, legal and illegal, proliferated, leading to gain for a few even while many lost much. In our unequal world, the nine top new billionaires gained a combined worth of $19.3 billion, enough to provide vaccines to more than three-fourths of a billion people in low-income countries. The pandemic was more than a public health issue; it had stunning and unsettling effects on our economic life. It raised questions about the role of the profit motive in supporting population health and about the degree to which corporate efforts should be supported by public money. It is now up to us to engage with these questions; to learn from the pandemic's economic effects; and to structure our economy to support a more just, equitable status quo, in which crises are occasions not for cashing in but, rather, for working together for the common good.

SECTION 4

EMOTIONS

OUR experience of health is inextricably linked to emotions. The feeling of health brings joy, freedom. The feeling of disease brings sadness, at times despair. COVID-19 delivered grief on a massive scale. Talking about health, particularly in the wake of a pandemic, means talking about emotions—and feeling them fully.

40

GRIEF AND LOSS

COVID-19 brought years of grief. More than 1 million Americans died from the disease, day after day, relentlessly. So much seemed precarious for so long. Grief swept through us. Multiplied across a country, individual griefs leave a great sadness. Grief is loss. What did we lose during COVID-19? Years of life, years of health, years of family time. Prolonged grief had the expected effects: depression, anxiety, cardiovascular decline. And we saw loss of jobs and income.

We also lost confidence. We could not control COVID-19. We looked for solace in uncertain science. We clung to changes in graphs and curves. With our data and models, we believed we could control and predict COVID-19. But the virus did not obey. We continued to reset our goals. We lived in uncertainty, and the humility suffering can bring.

We lost, for a time, our habits. We withdrew. We stayed indoors. Many of us were emotionally paralyzed, fearful. We were busy trying to survive. We did our work, cared for our children. We said goodbye on video screens. We watched funerals rather than attended them. Our rituals were interrupted.

Grief passes, though it can feel like it never will. The road through grief can lead to a radically transformed future. The

The Turning Point. Michael D. Stein and Sandro Galea, Oxford University Press.
© Oxford University Press 2024. DOI: 10.1093/oso/9780197749685.003.0040

time of COVID-19 was a truly remarkable period of movement-building; social change; and profound shifts in ideas, perspectives, and frameworks. Our COVID-19 grief merged somehow with centuries of racial grief, publicly experienced death by death. This caused us to emerge, for a time, from isolation, to protest against injustice.

"There is no love of life without despair of life," Albert Camus wrote. Grief pierced us, but will we change? From our present perspective of hindsight, we know where we are; where do we want to go? As we engage with this question, grief can be a clarifying influence. It shows us where we do not wish to return and suggests the way forward to a better future.

41

RECOGNIZING AND MOVING BEYOND OUR COLLECTIVE GRIEF

During the course of the COVID-19 pandemic, more than 1 million Americans died, and more than 6 million people died throughout the world. The dead are our family, friends, neighbors, colleagues, and all are mourned. Data suggest that 33 percent of Americans knew someone who died during these COVID-19 years; that would mean a total of approximately 100 million Americans grieved personal losses, grief that in and of itself had implications for health.

As we started to look past a global pandemic and move to rebuilding, the first step was recognizing the grief of many. This started with our personal lives, as we acknowledged and made space for sadness.

Beyond our individual sadness, the science on the mental health consequences of grief is sobering. A study conducted in 2014 showed that the bereavement period is linked with greater risk of new onset of multiple psychiatric disorders, regardless of when the grief happens during the life course. We already know that

The Turning Point. Michael D. Stein and Sandro Galea, Oxford University Press.
© Oxford University Press 2024. DOI: 10.1093/oso/9780197749685.003.0041

with COVID-19 there was a dramatic increase in anxiety or depressive disorders, with roughly four in 10 adults in the United States reporting symptoms early in the pandemic, an increase from one in 10 in January–June of 2019.

Recognizing that grief is almost certainly going to compound this psychological burden in the wake of large-scale tragedy is an important reminder of the burden of mental health need that we will face as a country in the wake of pandemics, one that could readily outstrip available services. This burden will have a long tail and will temporarily be overlooked; it was not newsworthy in the wake of the excitement over vaccines. But it will surely persist and reverberate across our schools and workplaces, and it suggests the need, once and finally, for a redoubling of our mental health resources. Importantly, we know that those who are marginalized and have fewer resources are bearing the greater burden of mental disorders, making it that much more important that we develop mental health services that are accessible to all. As always, the efforts of public health should focus first on helping the most vulnerable, engaging with the socioeconomic forces that create the context for their distress.

42

EPISTEMIC
HUMILITY DURING A
GLOBAL PANDEMIC

Much of this book has been about how challenging the COVID-19 years were for many people. Yet when we look beyond individual sorrows and losses, the COVID-19 moment has been, broadly speaking, good for public health as a discipline, and for many of the individuals working within it. During the pandemic, public health had visibility like never before, its central concerns in the headlines for more than a year. Prospective students applied to public health programs in record numbers. Epidemiologists were declared "the new rock stars" by *The New York Times*, and reporters wrote personal, human interest-oriented profiles of them—for example, asking them what they were doing for the holidays—holding the discipline up as a bellwether of data-informed good sense.

We, as a field, were delighted with this attention. Public health had long been overlooked in the public conversation, and seeing more interest in the profession was long overdue. It is, of course, also true that this heady moment held peril in that, during

The Turning Point. Michael D. Stein and Sandro Galea, Oxford University Press.
© Oxford University Press 2024. DOI: 10.1093/oso/9780197749685.003.0042

COVID-19, we ran the risk of overstating what we knew and the confidence with which we knew it, to the detriment of our field and its reputation.

One challenge has been our occasional lapses into false certitude. This is perhaps most clearly illustrated when we look back at the plethora of infectious disease models that emerged early and throughout the pandemic, all of which were fundamentally limited—as all models are—by the assumptions that informed them. We in the field well recognize the centrality of assumptions to model prediction—models are far better at explaining what happened than at predicting what might happen. But the declarative seriousness with which we presented some models throughout the pandemic at times contradicted our understanding of how they work.

Second, and relatedly, is the challenge of contradiction in our science. The paradigmatic example of this during COVID-19 concerns the utility of mask-wearing. In the early, acute phase of the pandemic, masking seemed clearly necessary. As the pandemic evolved, however, the benefits of masking in certain settings and among certain populations became less clear, engendering disagreement in public health about their continued use. Science is, of course, about learning and the refutation of past findings, about iteratively getting ever closer to the truth. But contradictions do not wear well when they are evolving in the public arena and accompanied by dispositive assertions that do not brook doubt. We should recognize how, when answers are evolving, disagreement can be useful, even essential.

Third, and also related, has been intolerance of disagreement in the field, reaching its zenith perhaps in the robust denunciation of efforts such as the Great Barrington Declaration, which recommended an approach to the pandemic that emphasized protecting the vulnerable while eschewing indefinite lockdowns. The Declaration, in its original formulation, embedded ideas that were contrary to mainstream views and could have been grounds for productive discussion and debate had there been space for it in our collective scientific conversation.

What unites these three concerns is epistemic arrogance, an overconfidence that may have been unavoidable in a moment of heightened regard for what we do. As we learn from the COVID-19 moment, it is perhaps time to re-embrace humility, to recalibrate, recognizing that what we know is always limited. In such moments, it is important to proceed with an openness to other points of view, embracing disagreement for its potential to be a constructive, clarifying influence. We will need to think together about how we can avoid the pitfalls of fame the next time we are cast quickly and harshly into the public eye.

43

THE SELLING OF VACCINES

During the summer of 2020, in what turned out to be a temporary lull in the COVID-19 pandemic before it hit again in full force in the fall, there was much discussion about the potential of the COVID-19 vaccines that were then in clinical trials. This included conversations about whether vaccines that had an efficacy of more than 50 percent would be sufficient for ending the crisis, and whether they should be recommended for widespread use. But then, in November 2020, we heard that not one, but two vaccines were more than 90 percent effective, and remarkably safe. This was extraordinary news and represented a true triumph of biomedical science, a reaping of reward for decades of investment, that surely promised a rapid end to the pandemic.

The vaccine euphoria extended to the widespread rollout of vaccines in early 2021, with many jostling for a place in line to receive the vaccine as quickly as possible. And vaccination rates in the United States rose quickly, pointing to a near future when all would be vaccinated. Until, of course, we hit a plateau. The early vaccine adopters all had their vaccine by the end of April, and the number of vaccines delivered in the United States slowed dramatically, with only half the population vaccinated. The vaccination

The Turning Point. Michael D. Stein and Sandro Galea, Oxford University Press.
© Oxford University Press 2024. DOI: 10.1093/oso/9780197749685.003.0043

effort pivoted quickly from trying to make sure there was enough supply to meet demand to puzzling over why there was not enough demand as supply flooded the country. Why were so many people hesitant to get a vaccine that was safe, potentially lifesaving, and free?

Much has since been written about vaccine hesitancy in the United States and globally, but, fundamentally, vaccine hesitancy during COVID-19 was shaped by trust—or, more precisely, by the lack of trust in a new, relatively untested medical intervention being delivered by a system that may not have inspired much trust in the past. We have long known that an important predictor of vaccine uptake is having a well-established health care provider whom one trusts. And the COVID-19 vaccination effort ran headlong into the limits of our trust in providers and the health system.

We also ran into the limits of the public's trust in public health. During the pandemic, we in public health essentially said "trust us" when it came to vaccines, and many initially did. Yet we saw the limits of this trust when we continued to say "trust us" with the same level of urgency for each new booster while the pandemic became less of a worry in the minds of many. Much of the public, even those who followed our recommendations closely earlier in the pandemic, simply said "no." It is clear that asking the public to follow our advice without providing new, data-informed reasons for why they should can lead to diminishing returns.

One can point to many causes for this lack of trust, but three reasons rise to the fore. First, we do not have a national comprehensive primary care system that allows Americans to develop long-term health care provider relationships. One-fourth of Americans do not have primary care providers; young adults have the least contact. The low value we place on preventive care and also difficulties with access caused by our fee-for-service payment models discourage such visits. Second, we have a long and sorry history of exclusion from the health care system felt by many groups, particularly communities of color. Third, we in public health do not always do the work of weighing the costs and benefits of certain measures before going all in on asking the public to embrace them. Often, our strategy is simply to say "take our word for it" and then hope for the best. The COVID-19 moment showed us that this approach is not enough. The next time, we will need to sharpen our thinking about how to better "sell" our recommendations to a sometimes rightly skeptical public.

44

WILL WE STOP BEING AFRAID?

The COVID-19 pandemic was terrifying, and understandably so. A disease that was unheard of in 2019 became the third leading cause of death in 2020 and was the leading cause of death in the United States in early 2021. The disease, transmitted through a respiratory virus, evoked horror movie tropes—we never knew whether we were close to someone who was infected, or even whether we ourselves might have been infected, spreading the disease to others.

We became afraid quickly, dramatically changing how we lived over the course of a few short weeks. We kept our distance from others, shifted workplace patterns, started wearing masks in public spaces, canceled our travel plans, and changed our minds about eating in restaurants. Fear of illness and death became a key predictor in our willingness to embrace measures to slow the spread of COVID-19. Fear was useful—it kept us safe, it saved lives, and it gave public health messages their emotional appeal.

Fear for our health was tolerable when we saw it as temporary, when we were looking forward to COVID-19 being over and we could simply undo the new ways of living and go back to

The Turning Point. Michael D. Stein and Sandro Galea, Oxford University Press.
© Oxford University Press 2024. DOI: 10.1093/oso/9780197749685.003.0044

life as we knew it in 2019. But it became clearer throughout 2021 as communities became vaccinated that the health risks from COVID-19 were never going to be completely over. This remains true today. SARS-CoV-2 is likely going to always be with us, at some baseline level.

Due to effective vaccines, the question has become: How do we mitigate fear in the face of still-present, albeit much-diminished, risk? We have to learn how to stop being afraid, or at least to live with our fear.

We have slowly lurched toward that learning. In the time since COVID-19, we have tried to identify and maintain some elements of the pandemic years to protect those who may be most vulnerable, while allowing life to resume, with human contact an ineluctable element of living. The undoing of fear involves our recalculation of risk and benefit. Should we keep masking forever in certain places such as airplanes? Do we want to maintain physical distancing norms in the places where we congregate? Should remote work remain a permanent fixture of our lives? What are the costs and benefits of keeping these measures in place? Now that we know COVID-19 will likely remain with us indefinitely in some form, we need to ask which features of pandemic life we wish to carry forward, shaping a new normal we can all live with.

45

HOPE DIES LAST

When COVID-19 hit the world, interest in the classic fictionalized account of a pandemic, Albert Camus' *The Plague*, soared, with sales more than tripling in the spring of 2020. Camus' book is keenly observant about human behavior in the face of contagion, with many lessons for our interaction with a modern pandemic. Toward the end of *The Plague*, Camus writes, "Once the faintest stirring of hope became possible, the dominion of the plague was ended." That captures the role that hope may play in ending a pandemic, but perhaps it is too simple a formulation. Hope does not just have a role to play at the end of a pandemic. Rather, it shapes our experience of the crisis all the way through.

We saw this during COVID-19. One of the features of the pandemic was its repeated waves of infection, spaced a few months apart. Infectious disease modeling had been limited in predicting what might happen after any given wave, leaving room for hope that each receding wave was the end of the pandemic, and that we could start dreaming of life with COVID-19 in the rearview mirror. The emergence of vaccines brought more hope, suggesting that we had the tools to push back the virus. This led to President Biden famously declaring a summer of freedom in 2021,

The Turning Point. Michael D. Stein and Sandro Galea, Oxford University Press.
© Oxford University Press 2024. DOI: 10.1093/oso/9780197749685.003.0045

only to see that envisioned idyll disrupted by yet another wave of infections across much of the United States, largely among persons who were unvaccinated. New viral mutations—first delta, then omicron—resulted in new waves, including among those who were vaccinated, reversing long hoped-for gains.

And yet, through wave after wave of the pandemic, we clung to hope. Perhaps hope is a necessary salve during such times, a life raft when the ship appears to be sinking. But, perhaps equally, we clung to hope because despite its pernicious and pervasive influence, COVID-19 never quite extinguished signs that we would get through it, despite the cost. Even as the economy reached record lows, governments intervened to create bailout packages that created bridges to an economic recovery in a post–COVID-19 world. And even as hundreds of thousands were infected by COVID-19, the majority of citizens were not.

Hope is different from optimism. Hope is grounded in context and reality. Optimism can be naive, without roots in a pragmatic vision of the world as it is. Hope is the persistent belief that the ultimate trajectory of events in their totality favors progress, and the emergence of a better world.

It is heartening to reflect that during COVID-19, even as the pandemic may have felt overwhelming, hope dared to insist upon itself, remaining a light amid darkness. Notably, this hope was made possible because we acted during COVID-19 to support the public good, because, flawed as it was, we *did* have a governmental response that aimed to mitigate the crushing impact of the pandemic. That is what kept hope alive. And it points to what we should invest in before the next pandemic hits us—the socioeconomic structures that sustain a healthier world.

46

CAN WE FORGET?

Approximately 1 million Americans died during the early
COVID-19 years. Mortality from a range of other diseases,
domestically and globally, also increased as behavioral health
risks rose and health care was stymied by efforts to contain the
pandemic. National life expectancy dropped nearly two years, its
largest decline since World War II. Efforts to contain COVID-19
ground the economy to a halt. Millions were suddenly unem-
ployed, in the most rapid downturn in employment ever seen in
the country, and nearly everyone found their working conditions
affected by COVID-19 in one way or another, from mask-wearing
to changes in patterns related to working from home or from the
office. Social life was similarly transformed by the pandemic,
first with the cancellation of essentially all indoor recreational
activities, and then with the emergence of rules governing social
engagements that had not existed as recently as 2019.

COVID-19 hit a country, and a world, that had essentially no
lived experience in how to cope with a large-scale global pandemic. Although previous pandemics of SARS and H1N1 were
harbingers of what was to come, they did not have a truly
global reach, and in no way prepared us for the sheer ubiq-
uity of the COVID-19 experience. COVID-19 seemed to affect

The Turning Point. Michael D. Stein and Sandro Galea. Oxford University Press.
© Oxford University Press 2024. DOI: 10.1093/oso/9780197749685.003.0046

everything—how we worked, how we played, where we lived, the supplies we were able to buy, the foods available to us, and the people we saw in the course of our day-to-day. As the pandemic receded, we were finally able to wonder: What would a world beyond COVID-19 look like? Would we forget the collective traumas of those three years?

In his poem "Once I Pass'd Through a Populous City," Walt Whitman writes of a woman he met: "Day by day and night by night we were together—all else has long been forgotten by me." Whitman's poetry reminds us of our own lives, for who has not been riveted by another person, an idea, or an object that blots out all else beyond the focus of our attention?

And this preoccupation, perhaps, holds a clue to what we might remember about COVID-19. Although COVID-19 was a global tragedy, it was a journey that all of us navigated through a set of individual experiences. What has become our lasting image or feeling—the haunting emptiness of buildings, the crushing loneliness of newly found time, the fear of infection, or the pain of losing loved ones? How have these experiences changed the way we live? Relatedly, what have we repressed or been unwilling to talk about? Answering these questions is the work of the present moment as we navigate this turning point and gain perspective on the trauma of the pandemic.

47

THE CENTRALITY
OF COMPASSION

A t the start of the COVID-19 pandemic, the national conversation centered around the notion that we were all at risk, that the pandemic "did not discriminate." It did not take long for us to realize how wrong that sentiment was. The pandemic did, in fact, discriminate, with persons of color and in low-wage jobs at greater risk of getting and dying from COVID-19. The disproportionate burden of COVID-19 on these groups—due both to greater risk of exposure and to greater underlying burden of preventable illness stemming from a history of more limited access to salutary resources—was as disquieting as it was predictable. If there is one canonical observation in all of health, it is that those who are marginalized and disadvantaged are going to be unhealthier than those who have access to more resources, particularly in times of crisis.

Why do we allow the world to be characterized by such health gaps? This answer is, in large part, in the way we think about these gaps. We continue to consider these health gaps to be inevitable, products of intractable social structures that we can do little about. And we absolve ourselves of responsibility for addressing them, expressing our willingness to do good largely through an

The Turning Point. Michael D. Stein and Sandro Galea. Oxford University Press.
© Oxford University Press 2024. DOI: 10.1093/oso/9780197749685.003.0047

empathetic embrace of charity. But empathy and charity rest on feeling others' pain. In being charitable, we can find ourselves seeing other people from afar, pitying them but not looking deeper into the structural causes of their distress. When we close ourselves off from recognizing the causes of the undue burden of poor health borne by others, our empathy and charity reach their limits. It then becomes acceptable for us to say that we have "done what we can." And what we can "do" is rarely enough.

Compassion offers a way past the limits of this approach. Motivated by awareness of our shared humanity, compassion compels us to ensure that all are healthy. Notably, it does not require us to feel others' pain. Rather, a compassionate approach pushes us to address the structural solutions—through civic engagement and investment—that can ensure that everyone is as healthy as possible. A compassionate understanding of the forces that generate poor health pushes us to see health as a public good, something that we all are invested in creating for one another.

How do we find the compassion to work to protect the health of all, particularly those who are different from us? Perhaps this requires a secular commitment to the values that bind us, health being central among them. Such a commitment can be catalyzed by tragedy, one that jolts us out of our usual way of seeing and doing things. Might COVID-19 represent such a moment? As the pandemic grows ever-more distant in our memory, it is important that we remember the lessons it taught us about compassion and work to apply them to our present-day approach to health.

48

FALSE CONFIDENCE

In 2009, President Obama declared a national emergency 11 days after the first case of swine flu was reported. Because recovery from the devastating Great Recession was the priority of the day, President Obama never shut down cities or businesses or schools. Republican governors and Congress fell in line quickly behind the Obama administration's health decisions, perhaps because the population most vulnerable to infection was children and those younger than age 30 years. Funding decisions faced little opposition. Epidemiologically, we got lucky. Swine flu turned out to be far less lethal than COVID-19.

We had been lucky before. While, in 2003, SARS resulted in the quarantine of thousands in Toronto, Canada, its effect was barely felt in the United States. Other outbreaks such as Ebola seemed far away and barely touched our shores.

This good fortune perhaps left us with a false sense of confidence about our ability to weather pandemics. That false sense of confidence may have been disastrous in the context of COVID-19.

The Trump administration waited 53 days after the first case of COVID-19 was detected in the United States to declare a national emergency. During those weeks, the president himself declared the virus "is going to disappear" like "a miracle." The Centers for

The Turning Point. Michael D. Stein and Sandro Galea, Oxford University Press.
© Oxford University Press 2024. DOI: 10.1093/oso/9780197749685.003.0048

Disease Control and Prevention were demoralized and silenced. The threat was dismissed.

Soon, we were faced with a highly contagious, lethal virus, with few medical tools at our disposal. We had only the tools of public health. And this time, our infection surveillance—the first tool of public health—was particularly poor after decades of underinvestment. This set the stage for a catastrophically poor national response, until we were saved by astonishingly effective vaccines.

This begs the question: How much of our failure was due to our overconfidence, informed by recent outbreaks that turned out to be not overly consequential? And how much of that overconfidence could have been averted by a more honest reckoning with our vulnerabilities, and by the effort that would have been required to combat a really lethal pandemic in the years leading up to COVID-19?

Although COVID-19 was much worse than swine flu biologically, the truth is we still got lucky with it. Mortality from SARS is 10 percent, that from MERS is 34 percent, and that from H7N9 bird flu is more than 39 percent—respiratory viruses all far more deadly than COVID-19. Fortune may have favored us during the pandemic years, but it will not do so forever. We should prepare now for that inevitable day.

49

A TALE OF VOLITION

Groups long marginalized by health systems continue to have limited access to vaccines. This is heartbreaking—a moral failure. But what about groups whose vaccination is curtailed by personal choice rather than by structural factors? As many as one-third of the U.S. population could have been vaccinated easily against COVID-19 but simply did not want to be. How should we understand their vaccine refusal?

Herman Melville's 1853 short story, "Bartleby, the Scrivener," reckons with the possibility that freedom can be realized through a refusal to submit. Bartleby is the hardworking, dutiful scribe of a Wall Street lawyer, who, at a certain point, refuses to do the tasks that his life demands. When he is asked to do his job, he responds, "I would prefer not to." Thereafter, he refuses everything, eventually even food and water, until he dies of starvation.

"I would prefer not to" haunts the story because Bartleby offers no reason for his refusal. We want to know *why* he would prefer not to, but there is no reason given. He does not need to give a reason.

By contrast, COVID-19 vaccine refusers offered many reasons in 2021, the first full year of vaccine availability. They often claimed

The Turning Point. Michael D. Stein and Sandro Galea. Oxford University Press.
© Oxford University Press 2024. DOI: 10.1093/oso/9780197749685.003.0049

there was not yet enough real-world experience of the vaccine's safety (despite hundreds of millions of doses administered). They said any new vaccine could have produced late side effects we did not know about. Or they said that COVID-19 was mostly a mild disease, or that they would be fortunate or careful enough to avoid infection. But none of these reasons are in and of themselves sufficient explanation.

A century and a half after its creation, Melville's story still holds an unsettling truth about some of our neighbors: There is self-gratification in refusal. COVID-19 revealed the inexplicable, powerful, triumphant feeling that we all have the ability to opt out, even against our better judgment. It looks like madness, and perhaps it is, "but it is *my* madness," the unvaccinated person may think. The simple refusal to act on behalf of one's obvious self-interest is defiance, and, to some, defiance is courage. Bartleby's emphatic and unexplained "no" was an act of volition, life-affirming in a way. Likewise, in 2021, Americans had several vaccine choices, but they could do exactly as they pleased, even if it led to self-destruction. The unvaccinated likely felt entitled to this freedom, as a fundamental right.

But in this case, it was not so simple. During COVID-19, we were inextricably bound to neighbors who, while disregarding what was obviously in their own best interest, compromised the best interests of others. For the vaccinated, attempts at self-defense—with distancing, with masks—had not been enough; the robust protection of vaccines needed to be widely accepted to keep COVID-19 manageable. Should we then have required the vaccine everywhere? Making vaccination a requirement for military service, entry to schools, workplaces, airplanes, even gyms and restaurants would have increased the number of vaccinated people in the United States and moved everyone closer to the life they remembered from before 2020. But it would also have taken away the autonomy of refusal for the increasingly few who would have preferred not to have their wishes denied.

50

TRUST AND COVID-19

A key feature of pandemics is their capacity to test our notions of collective trust. In the fearful era of COVID-19, we were asked to trust in government, in institutions, and in each other. For nearly two years, we tested whether trust is a sine qua non in a public health crisis. In some ways, we failed this test, but in other ways there may be reasons for optimism.

Sixty years ago, the vast majority of Americans had faith in government. Today, roughly the same majority say they do not. But it is worth remembering that even during Reagan's years in office, trust in the presidency never rose above 45 percent of the public; it has sunk steadily since, regardless of president or party. In the 2020s, however, it seems to have hit a new low: Many do not even trust elections.

Perhaps most worrisome for efforts to bring about effective immunity that could mitigate the spread of a pandemic, a 2021 poll found only 52 percent of Americans really trusted the Centers for Disease Control and Prevention; the numbers for state and local health departments were even lower. During COVID-19, town meetings turned into battlegrounds where public health officials were sometimes physically threatened; more than 500 left their jobs as the pandemic progressed. As the requirement of

The Turning Point. Michael D. Stein and Sandro Galea, Oxford University Press.
© Oxford University Press 2024. DOI: 10.1093/oso/9780197749685.003.0050

trust has broadened from the everyday realm of direct personal relationships to faith in more abstract entities—governments, public health departments, scientific authorities—the bonds of trust have frayed.

COVID-19 revealed the extent of our distrust. We distrusted our fellow citizens. We feared that our privacy would be invaded. We wanted to control our personal information. The management of the pandemic was shadowed by conspiracy, doubt, and hesitancy. COVID-19 did not create social glue; there was no common purpose. We were cynical about each other's motives.

Yet, in some ways, it was a good few years for trust. Researchers throughout the world shared genomic sequences, epidemiological insights, and early clinical trial results faster than at any time in the past. Accepting the lockdown was an altruistic activity, agreed to by most people in high-risk areas. The financial fallout of COVID-19, affecting the most vulnerable among us, was softened by bipartisan federal legislation, a rare achievement. In a world tuned to the frequency of distrust, such movements are hopeful indeed.

Still, as public health certainties were undermined, trust in public health declined, and frustration sometimes crept into official pronouncements, with "trust us" becoming animated by the subtext, "do as we say." This continued to harm trust, and public health has not yet fully regained the public's confidence. There are no shortcuts to getting it back. Trust must be earned.

SECTION 5

THE FUTURE

COVID-19 was a tragedy. But it was also a turning point that can direct us toward a better future. What will that future look like? What steps can we take in the present to ensure it is as healthy as it can be? How we engage with these questions will determine whether we seize the opportunities of this moment to shape a radically healthier nation.

51

THE NEW US?

History teaches that population-wide behavioral patterns change infrequently and slowly. After all, little changed in how we behaved after the last global disease disruption, the flu pandemic of 1968, and, perhaps most dramatically, societal behavioral changes after the 1918 flu pandemic were few and far between. What is most striking about how we act in the present is how similar our behavior looks to what it was like in the past.

What did change after the 1918 flu pandemic was our appreciation of the need to move beyond considering health as an exclusively individual responsibility and to set up the structures needed to help promote health collectively. A number of countries created health ministries after the 1918 pandemic and centralized health care delivery schemes, which unfolded in different ways in different nations. Russia, for example, was first to follow the 1918 flu pandemic with public health care, funded through state-run insurance. The United Kingdom, France, and Germany did much the same soon after. In 1922, the League of Nations Health Committee and Health Sections were established, forerunners of the World Health Organization.

This teaches us that crisis can create an opportunity for change, but that change is unlikely to be sustained purely through

The Turning Point. Michael D. Stein and Sandro Galea. Oxford University Press improvements in individual behavior. Somewhat like New Year's resolutions—eagerly made, just as quickly broken—individual behavior change is evanescent. What large-scale traumas such as the COVID-19 pandemic create an opportunity for is system-wide change that can, over time, have a slow, but critical, influence on collective human behavior. This means that as we look back on the pandemic years, we have an opportunity to be deliberate about what those changes could be. What will our post–COVID-19 legacy look like? Will we finally recognize that having millions of people without ready access to affordable health care exposes them, and all of us, to the worst consequences of infectious disease, and that the United States needs guaranteed health insurance for all? Will we better fund public health agencies so that they have the resources to tackle novel infectious disease outbreaks? Will we finally realign our decision-making processes so that we recognize that all policies—from transportation to finance, housing, and the environment—matter for health?

It would be a pity not to use this moment to create a better world; our effort to do so may be more fruitfully focused on how to build the structures that support such a world rather than on trying, in vain, to change human nature around the choices we make about health.

52

WHO DECIDES?

The COVID-19 moment has been fraught with countless arguments about the trade-offs between strict measures to control viral contagion and the economic consequences of these trade-offs. At the heart of these arguments has been one—often unspoken—question: Who gets to decide what is right for societies? Who decides how to evaluate the trade-offs? Perhaps these questions are best illuminated by analogy. Increases in speed limits throughout the United States have been associated with 37,000 deaths over 25 years. In 1993, 41 states had a maximum speed limit of 65 miles per hour (mph); the other nine states had a speed limit of 55 mph. In the early 2020s, by contrast, 41 states had maximum speed limits of 70 mph or higher; six had 80 mph speed limits. The change happened slowly, as advocacy groups argued for higher speed limits to reflect the reality that many drivers exceed the speed limit anyway.

The trade-offs here appear to be clear. A 5 mph increase in maximum speed limit is associated with an eight percent increase in interstate fatalities; it also saves a bit more than six minutes on a 100-mile trip when driving at 70 mph versus 65 mph. Is the

The Turning Point. Michael D. Stein and Sandro Galea. Oxford University Press.
© Oxford University Press 2024. DOI: 10.1093/oso/9780197749685.003.0052

increased risk of death worth the thrill of driving faster and saving time on travel?

We know that reducing speed limits to levels that are still quite fast—65 mph—will save lives. The highway speed limit in Canada, for example, is 100 kilometers per hour (approximately 62 mph); the motor vehicle fatality rate per capita in Canada is also approximately half what it is in the United States.

Prevention is at the core of public health. We know what we should do, because we know that lowering speed limits saves lives.

But we have long accepted, as a society, that public health does not get to decide what speed limits should be. That decision ultimately rests with elected officials, or regulatory agencies appointed by those officials. Why? Groups of elected officeholders are the only bodies within society that are directly accountable to the populations affected by the rules they set. It is on them to balance trade-offs, to listen to the input from public health, but also to listen to the input from enthusiasts for higher speeds who value their freedom to go faster. And if elected officials miscalibrate the trade-offs, they can be held accountable for their actions by being removed from office.

Such political decisions are, to be sure, open to particular manipulation by special interest groups, including motor vehicle manufacturers that may have sales and profits to gain from vehicles going fast, even as they suffer few direct consequences. But our democratic system is designed to give voice to competing ideas and values, within a pluralist world.

The voice of public health clearly should be central in decision-making around policies affecting the well-being of populations. But even in a pandemic, our role is not to dictate policy; rather, we should be the best possible advocates for an approach that values life and health above all else. Fundamentally, we have a critical—and singular—perspective, one that should be heard. However, it is ultimately up to society to decide how it wants to structure itself, through the offices of our elected representatives.

53

FIXING OUR HEALTH
SYSTEM AFTER COVID-19

The COVID-19 pandemic was the best of times and the worst of times for our health care system. We saw the ceaseless and effective efforts of frontline doctors and nurses as they worked to contain an unprecedented plague. Yet we also were reminded of the fragility of our medical system, as we saw it buckling at times under the weight of a new disease, made worse by lack of access to quality care for many and a population burdened by chronic diseases that made COVID so much worse.

The pandemic made even clearer what we have long known: Our health care system matters. How do we protect it? Three ideas come to mind.

First, we can adopt payment models that incentivize health rather than sickness. We currently have a model that incentivizes providing ever-more expensive care for disease. Rather than being a health care system, it is, in truth, a sick care system. We readily treat people who are sick; we are less skilled at improving health across entire populations so that people do not get sick in the first place. Changing incentives means embedding public health practices within our health care system.

The Turning Point. Michael D. Stein and Sandro Galea, Oxford University Press.
© Oxford University Press 2024. DOI: 10.1093/oso/9780197749685.003.0053

Second, health care professionals need to engage with the social forces that shape health. We can do this by incorporating foundational factors into medical education. During medical school interviewing courses, doctors have traditionally been taught to take family and social histories. An even wider focus on the forces that produce health—clean air, nutritious food, safe neighborhoods, and livable wages—can provide the perspective that lets doctors truly support health rather than just treat disease. Clinicians can see themselves throughout their careers as being part of the architecture that generates patients' health rather than playing a role only when patients are sick. A deeper understanding of our complex world can be accelerated by cultivating a more diverse population of physicians. How might care be better for people of color, for example, if more doctors understood the Black experience from having lived it?

Third, health care providers can use their public voices to change the narrative about health. This means communicating the link between socioeconomic forces and prevention. Providers can tell the full story of health—not just the story of medical care. We saw, during COVID-19, how one of the most powerful forces shaping the narrative was individual doctors speaking about their experiences. It is time for doctors to speak routinely about the full range of social factors that shape their patients' lives.

We want an excellent health care system—we all want outstanding doctors and nurses to look after us when we are sick. But to prevent ourselves from living shorter, sicker lives, we need more than a health care system—we need a system that actually generates health. And we need it long before the next pandemic strikes.

54

HIV AND COVID-19

Two pandemics bookend the past 40 years: HIV and COVID-19. The first changed our view of health care and its delivery in dramatic ways. Perhaps the second will—once the passage of time has given us the same perspective on it that we now have on HIV—change our view of health and who has access to it.

Three years after the initial 1981 publication of a report on persons with a new infectious syndrome, activist Larry Kramer wrote an article titled "1,112 and Counting," in which he berated every government official connected with health care—from the Centers for Disease Control and Prevention (CDC) and the National Institutes of Health (NIH) administrators to local politicians—for refusing to acknowledge the widening AIDS epidemic (President Reagan had not yet said the word "HIV" publicly and would not for four more years). The burden of HIV fell on certain marginalized groups. As the HIV epidemic surged, gay men demanded vigorous federal intervention on their behalf. They wanted the benefits, protections, and resources that only the federal government could provide. Cohesive activism slowly developed, taking years to organize. Its reshaping of public opinion around HIV and biomedical activities eventually produced dramatic results. The average U.S. Food and

The Turning Point. Michael D. Stein and Sandro Galea, Oxford University Press.
© Oxford University Press 2024. DOI: 10.1093/oso/9780197749685.003.0054

Drug Administration approval time of new drugs went from a decade to a year. Patient groups had to be consulted when new drugs were being reviewed by federal agencies. The purity of the placebo-controlled trial was reimagined. Consumers started to demand to know treatment options and success rates and to be able to shop for the best care. It was a new era in biomedicine and in being a patient in the health care system.

Let us now jump ahead 40 years. The political response to COVID-19's arrival was in some ways worse than Reagan's choice to ignore AIDS. On January 2, 2020, the director of the CDC contacted the National Security Council to warn about early cases of the coronavirus in China and the potential that it could spread to the United States. Yet when President Trump's first televised remarks about it came three weeks later, he said, "We have it totally under control. It's one person coming in from China, and we have it under control. It's going to be just fine." Warnings by scientists were soon termed a "hoax." The disinformation campaign that followed mattered because COVID-19, a respiratory illness, was a broader threat to the general public than HIV ever was.

Unlike with HIV, we watched our health care infrastructure become overloaded by persons with COVID-19, and we saw thousands of health care workers die. Yet our experience of this pandemic was not shaped by an activist group attacking the health care system or its governing institutions. After all, the NIH and its pharmaceutical company collaborators developed miraculous vaccines with astounding speed and hospital workers did the best they could.

Vaccines, however, require vaccination; biomedicine becomes prevention via distribution through public health channels. During the pandemic, we witnessed the problems of delivery of this form of preventive care, with thousands of Americans dying each day while vaccines sat in warehouses or were inequitably delivered. As production of vaccines ramped up, they were delivered on an old-fashioned medical schedule; few vaccination centers ran around the clock, seven days a week.

How will the experience of COVID-19 reshape the working of public health, as HIV did? What are the benefits and protections that government can provide going forward, as we face the risk of new pandemics? Will we widen insurance coverage to all Americans? Will we address the structural inequalities that produced high COVID-19 vulnerability among Black Americans, essential workers, the poor, and those living in rural communities? COVID-19 has not evidenced the need for a change simply in health care delivery but, rather, in how we think of health more generally. This means a new conceptualization of public health and what we are owed as citizens. HIV was a tragedy, but at least we can say we learned from it and applied these lessons to creating positive, fundamental change. Will we be able to say the same about COVID-19?

55

GUNS AND THE UNANTICIPATED CONSEQUENCES OF COVID-19

The pandemic brought many unanticipated consequences, from the health effects of lockdowns to the unpredictable course of the disease itself, with its many symptoms and variants. Then there was how it intersected, in sometimes surprising ways, with long-standing social and political issues, such as the challenge of gun violence, which intensified during COVID-19. In 2020, even with much of the population staying at home, the number of mass shootings exceeded the year-end totals of the previous five years. With 20,000 dead from guns, COVID-19 did not slow the gun violence trend of the past decade. In frequency, fatalities, and injuries, gun violence continued to take a toll on the United States.

Far from seeing gun violence abate during the pandemic, 2020 was, in many ways, the year of the gun in America. It was a year that saw the highest gun sales ever. There were 2 million guns sold in March 2020 alone, making the month that COVID-19 rates first rose the second busiest month for gun sales in history. This rise

The Turning Point. Michael D. Stein and Sandro Galea, Oxford University Press.
© Oxford University Press 2024. DOI: 10.1093/oso/9780197749685.003.0055

in sales was largely driven by first-time buyers. Americans feared crime waves, police depletion, and government repression—and sales reflected this. Americans stockpiled military weapons and high-volume gun clips. The background check system foundered in the face of record-breaking business. Notably, the number of recorded gun sales included only *known* gun sales; sales of unregistered guns, those bought at gun fairs, and online "ghost guns" assembled by the purchaser were not tracked. But shootings continued, related to factors such as criminal activity, family disputes, and gang wars. Despite widespread desire to ensure protection through gun ownership, 2020 was yet another year when more gun sales did not buy more safety. Following the pandemic year, we continued to see the mass shootings that have become a uniquely American phenomenon. This included the school shooting in Uvalde, Texas, in which 19 children and two adults were killed.

Then there were other kinds of shootings, those that are less talked about: suicides committed with a firearm. When the pandemic struck, suicide by gun had been on the rise for years, and COVID-19—with its economic disruption, bleak joblessness, and enforced isolation—brought new pressures to a nation already armed and despairing. Making matters more difficult, stay-at-home orders curtailed outreach by mental health workers and social programs that might have ameliorated the growing violence.

This rise in gun violence in 2020 was a continuation from 2019; that is, it preceded the effects of the pandemic and the summer of unrest that followed the killing of George Floyd. This reminds us that neither racial issues nor a novel infectious disease necessarily worsened the problem of American gun violence. Although the rise in gun violence during COVID-19 reflects the difficulty of anticipating the effects of large-scale traumatic events such as a pandemic, it is also true that there are root causes that keep gun violence in circulation in our society. We cannot, then, ascribe gun violence to anything fleeting or unprecedented. When we look at this problem, we are looking, fundamentally, at ourselves, at the needless death we continue to accept. There is no escaping the fact that engaging with this challenge means addressing its deeply rooted social and political causes. Although there is evidence for many policies that can reduce fatalities—such as assault weapons and large-capacity magazine bans—we need to intervene both through new policy action around gun safety and by addressing the issue's cultural underpinnings. Until we address these root causes, the country will remain febrile and trigger ready. A healthier future depends on our willingness to confront this urgent American problem.

56

POLICIES THAT PERSIST

Alcohol sales, particularly sales of hard liquor, increased in 2020 more than in any year in two decades. The closing of bars drove alcohol consumption lower during the first spring of COVID-19, but by summer the liquor laws had changed in 39 states, allowing income-deprived establishments to sell alcohol to go. Now we could walk to the corner restaurant or bar and carry out alcohol. To-go purchases bypassed prior concerns among legislators (and public health leaders) about fostering underage drinking and intoxicated driving. Restaurants got into the game, acquiring new liquor licenses. Alcohol was also delivered in new ways. Uber bought the company Drizly so anyone could order cocktails with a telephone call and have their drink of choice driven to their door a half hour later. It was suddenly just easier to obtain liquor everywhere. The updated laws were a business "success," producing new revenue streams for restaurant owners who had lost diners and for entrepreneurial bars, saving businesses and jobs. Not since the end of Prohibition had the rules about alcohol changed so abruptly and significantly. The public health concerns that were originally behind limiting alcohol-to-go sales were overridden by economic need.

The Turning Point. Michael D. Stein and Sandro Galea, Oxford University Press.
© Oxford University Press 2024. DOI: 10.1093/oso/9780197749685.003.0056

Perhaps not surprisingly, following this change of laws, drinking across the population increased. The largest increase occurred among those who lost jobs. Drinking among women notably increased from pre-pandemic levels. Under lockdown, alcohol use disorder and dependence flourished. Good economics had bad health consequences. Because alcohol is an immune system suppressant as well as a potent behavioral risk inducer, it likely made drinkers more vulnerable to COVID-19. More directly, heavier drinking produced more liver disease and more domestic violence during the COVID-19 years.

Was the loosening of restrictions on alcohol-to-go sales during COVID-19 a reasonable balance of economic interests with health interests? That question will likely be debated for some time. The debate is particularly pointed because it involves small businesses, the centerpieces of most communities. In a divided political world, alcohol regulatory change had received bipartisan support, making the "success" story of changing alcohol regulations particularly noteworthy.

As the pandemic wound its way to an end, 20 states decided to maintain their laws allowing takeaway alcohol, despite the ongoing health risk. Should we have had these purchasing accommodations in the first place? Do we value easy access to alcohol so much that we should be willing to pay a higher health price in terms of its consequences?

These are the questions that we ask all the time when we make decisions to limit harmful products or behavior. The COVID-19 moment caused us to rush many of these decisions without much deliberation. It is now up to us to think more carefully about how we want to organize our world and what price we are willing to pay for risky, but perhaps enjoyable, behaviors such as drinking alcohol.

THE INVISIBLE WORK
OF PUBLIC HEALTH

A mid the devastation caused by COVID-19, the Biden administration allocated $7.4 billion to hire public health workers, infusing the public health system with resources. The new funding was designed to put state and local health departments on stronger financial footing to engage with both the long list of public health projects that existed before COVID-19 and the work necessary to mitigate the pandemic. These goals notwithstanding, how any individual health department uses funds is always uncertain. Now that we have faced COVID-19, how have we done in returning to a wider view of the priorities of public health? Indeed, it is worth asking, Do most Americans even know much about the work of public health outside the context of COVID-19?

During the pandemic, Americans were given a very particular idea of what public health work involves based on COVID-19, which dominated news reports for years. This idea involves conducting rapid case identification and tracing contacts for additional COVID-19 testing; isolation of cases and quarantine of close contacts; and epidemiologists creating databases for disease surveillance, risk factor assessment, disease mapping, and making policy recommendations. Beyond these pandemic-related

The Turning Point. Michael D. Stein and Sandro Galea, Oxford University Press
© Oxford University Press 2024. DOI: 10.1093/oso/9780197749685.003.0057

activities, most Americans have likely forgotten—or never even known—what public health practitioners do.

Most people have of course heard of the Centers for Disease Control and Prevention (CDC), the federally funded flagship institution of public health. But many do not realize that local health departments are the front lines of a federal, state, and local partnership. Do most citizens know that state and local public health work includes wellness promotion, environmental oversight, safe workplace checks, restaurant inspection, programs for mothers and infants, childhood vaccinations, HIV outreach, rabies control, tobacco use and obesity reduction campaigns, economic and policy analysis around delivering and evaluating health, or assisting communities in disaster preparedness? It is doubtful most people know that thousands of nurses and physicians are employed by health departments or that the activities of individual health departments vary throughout the country.

Perhaps more important, does the public recognize that one of the factors that contributed to our lack of COVID-19 preparedness was that we had been starving our public health infrastructure of funds for the first two decades of the 21st century? This begs the question: Did our disinvestment in public health before COVID-19 reflect our disinterest in funding the historically wide assortment of public health work? Or did our disinvestment simply reflect ignorance about how essential public health infrastructure is to our health? We live in a moment when the operationalization of the government's duty to protect the public has been questioned, when we do not trust health agencies, including the CDC. As the pandemic fades, it is time to reconsider our values and to ask what we really want our public health infrastructure to do—and then to fund it accordingly.

58

WILL BETTER PUBLIC HEALTH FUNDING BE ENOUGH?

By 2020, public health system funding had decreased per population older than age 30 years due to a combination of budgetary decisions and population growth. At that time, most U.S. states spent less than $100 per person on public health, and most local governments spent more on policing than on health. There had been warnings about the state of public health funding and calls to expand our public health infrastructure for at least a decade, yet the public health system entered the pandemic down more than 20 percent of its workforce capacity.

It is clear that when COVID-19 arrived, public health was underfunded. It is worth asking, If public health departments had been fully funded, would the pandemic have gone differently, reducing the extent of death and morbidity?

Although the United States had encountered transmissible infections several times in the past, it is certainly difficult to prepare for a once-in-a-century pandemic. A better resourced public health system might have invested in improved strategic capacity-building: information technology to share data, replacement of

The Turning Point. Michael D. Stein and Sandro Galea, Oxford University Press.
© Oxford University Press 2024. DOI: 10.1093/oso/9780197749685.003.0058

antiquated computers, more thoughtful integration of local and state data sharing, and an updated disease reporting system. In parallel, health departments might have invested in different programs or maintained a larger workforce—keeping trained contact tracers in place, for example, or more laboratory personnel to develop novel viral detection methods.

All these steps would have been an improvement on the status quo. Yet, would a better funded public health system have been able to respond as robustly to COVID-19 as we would have liked? The answer is, it is complicated. The public health system in the United States is decentralized. Despite the Centers for Disease Control and Prevention's preeminence, public health authority belongs not only to the 50 states but also to thousands of counties and municipalities. This patchwork structure necessarily produces intergovernmental conflicts, delays and gaps in data collection, and can undermine the authority of public health officials seeking to create blanket rules.

This decentralization affected all aspects of the response to COVID-19. Immunizations, for example, may be provided by a local health department in one region but by other entities (e.g., pharmacies) in a second region. Thus, immunization, considered by many an essential public health program, was not rolled out according to a national model. If it had been, could we have vaccinated more people, faster?

Over and above the role of the public health system, it is worth noting that it was aspects of American society—which lay outside the scope of public health department activities—that made the U.S. population susceptible to the rapid community spread and mounting deaths of COVID-19. Health departments did not focus on the provision of better care for the elderly or on structural inequalities that produced high vulnerability among essential workers, two key constituencies that drove the U.S. epidemic. It will take constant attention to, and investment in, improving the foundational drivers of health to truly mitigate the risk of another pandemic, but public health has historically not been empowered to tackle these issues.

There is little question that we need to better fund our public health infrastructure. But doing so will not be enough to prevent the next pandemic. We also need to think about the organization of our public health systems and the full scope of the forces that create health. Early thinking on this front will require a collective reconsideration of the roles and activities of public health institutions.

59

CHRONIC COVID

Influenza in its worst seasons produces millions of cases and tens of thousands of American deaths. In this way, it is not unlike COVID-19. But one of COVID-19's additional threats, differentiating it from influenza, is the ongoing set of health problems that COVID-19 infection, even mild infection, may produce—so-called long COVID.

Long COVID has become the familiar name for what is wrong with persons who have a constellation of symptoms—shortness of breath, fatigue, chest pain, brain fog, muscle aches, dizziness, and memory loss—that continue after initial infection, more scientifically named post-acute sequelae of SARS-CoV-2. This syndrome affects approximately one in 12 of those who have had COVID-19 infection, and it seems to be more common if the initial infection was severe. But the definition of long COVID varies, and we are still in the process of determining its causes. Is long COVID an autoimmune process or the result of viral persistence in the body or is it psychosomatic—the result of the fear, anxiety, and grief that were the hallmarks of the pandemic years? We know of other acute infections that sometimes lead to chronic symptoms—Lyme disease, for example, and Epstein–Barr virus. Yet such chronicity is relatively rare. In addition, we know of other novel respiratory

The Turning Point. Michael D. Stein and Sandro Galea, Oxford University Press.
© Oxford University Press 2024. DOI: 10.1093/oso/9780197749685.003.0059

RNA viruses that cause acute symptoms and, in a subset of patients, produce an assortment of persistent nonrespiratory symptoms. For example, one-fourth of SARS survivors had chronic fatigue years later. Other RNA viruses, such as Ebola, have also produced long-term health consequences. However, because its pathology is unclear, because of its diverse manifestations, because it does not kill or hospitalize, and because there are no treatments, doubt has characterized the conversation about long COVID from the very beginning.

All chronic illnesses are depressing for sufferers. But are long COVID symptoms caused by depression or vice versa? Even if the cause (or causes) is unknown, patients want their illnesses named. A diagnosis is a starting point for conversation, an admission that something is wrong.

Linked to the mass traumatic event of a pandemic, the uncertain scale of long COVID bothers us because it carries a particular cultural question: What can we overcome and what may protractedly affect us? We have seen a new infectious disease pass among us, causing chaos in our economic and social systems. Which of these disruptions can be cured and which will be long-lasting?

Like so much else in the COVID-19 era, there is new information about long COVID accumulating all the time, even if most evidence is not definitive, and we are still not confident of our answers. COVID-19 has taught that it takes time and many mistakes to understand the effects of new pathogens, suggesting that the truth about long COVID will take years to emerge.

60

COVID-19 COLLECTIVISM

Millions may have developed long COVID during 2020 in the year before we had vaccines. Post-vaccine, as COVID-19 became endemic and less lethal, many more were in a position to develop long-lasting symptoms, creating a growing public health concern. Science remains uncertain about the cause and character of the post-acute sequelae of SARS-CoV-2, and the biological factors that may contribute to the condition remain unknown. Nearly half of all initial COVID-19 infections are asymptomatic, and, as best as we understand for the time being, long-lasting symptoms are particularly diffuse. All this suggests that it is going to take a large number of patients enrolled in rigorous studies to help us better understand long COVID in the coming years.

Forty years after HIV/AIDS changed many patients into the partners of academic researchers in the hunt for new treatments, long COVID patients are coming together with a new generation of scientists to drive discovery. For example, the advocacy group Survivor Corps is a grassroots organization that has mobilized its members to support scientific research. Following early anecdotal reports that vaccines may offer relief to some people with long COVID symptoms, Survivor Corps surveyed members and found that 45 percent of respondents indeed reported some form of

The Turning Point. Michael D. Stein and Sandro Galea, Oxford University Press.
© Oxford University Press 2024. DOI: 10.1093/oso/9780197749685.003.0060

symptom resolution after vaccination. These results led to a more formal, carefully monitored longitudinal study. Patient groups can make important observations, help with patient recruitment into clinical trials and other research opportunities, and provide platforms for data harmonization. The Long COVID Alliance promotes the central tenet of patient self-advocacy: "Nothing about us, without us."

Some long COVID patient collectives provide online support groups to decrease the isolation of chronic illness. Others have a policy focus, fostering public–private partnerships or advancing health equity. Scientific and patient advocacy groups have joined in calls for government investment in long COVID research and were rewarded in 2021 when the National Institutes of Health launched a $1.15 billion initiative to study long COVID, which researchers and patients hope will provide biological answers and ensure that the odd and lingering symptoms of long COVID are not dismissed as psychogenic illness.

The scale of long COVID will likely create a new public health crisis with the rise of a novel disability, often affecting young adults, that will require resources and thoughtful policies. We will need the expertise of specialists and an attitude that permits patients to drive research directions, informed by a concern for the collective good.

61

CAN WE BE LED?

On March 13, 2020, President Trump declared a national emergency due to the COVID-19 pandemic. The country scrambled to adapt, with workplaces that could afford to have their employees work from home shifting nearly overnight to remote work. We remember that shift distinctly, and we also remember how we thought, at the time, that we would be able to return to work within a few weeks. But, of course, COVID-19 did not let up in the spring of 2020. The original national emergency declaration, Proclamation 9994, was renewed by President Biden a year after the original declaration. With each wave of the pandemic receding, it seemed as though the virus was ebbing, only for another wave to remind us that SARS-CoV-2 was still circulating. President Biden's 2021 "summer of freedom," buoyed by optimism about the potential of the COVID-19 vaccines, fell substantially short of the mark as the pandemic raged among those who were unvaccinated. This led to us coming to grips with the recognition that COVID-19 would likely be with us, in endemic form, for the foreseeable future.

Perhaps naively, we were once interested in when the virus would stop circulating, bringing about the end of the pandemic. Then our focus shifted from the evolving set of behaviors we adopted

The Turning Point. Michael D. Stein and Sandro Galea, Oxford University Press.
© Oxford University Press 2024. DOI: 10.1093/oso/9780197749685.003.0061

to protect ourselves from a pandemic emergency to a steady state of behaviors that continued to manage risk while allowing us to get on with our lives. This was an important conceptual shift, moving us from waiting for the risk from the virus to be "over" to recognizing that we will always have some risk and asking what steps we were willing to take to mitigate that risk.

The question then becomes, In the wake of a pandemic, which measures are we going to carry forward—such as face coverings in crowded areas, home testing for infectious diseases, and telehealth—and which will we consign to history?

It seems reasonable that two principles should guide us in this consideration. First, the presence of an ongoing threat must be balanced by the need to live full lives, to ensure that the world moves forward, that future generations have the opportunities that were available to earlier ones. This means that we have a responsibility to preserve—even if it comes with some risk—the behaviors that create those opportunities. For instance, we need to promote ways to safely gather, to interact with each other and our communities.

Second, we must protect those who are most at risk for severe disease. Our early responses to COVID-19 were not risk stratified. Nearly all adopted masking behaviors, and nearly all institutions shut down—including schools, despite the lower risk experienced by children. But we now know clearly that it was persons who were aged 65 years or older, or who had reasons for immunosuppression, who were at greater risk and that mitigation should have been primarily aimed at protecting those who bore this elevated risk. This includes properly protecting those whose work put them in greatest contact with a new infectious disease.

As we emerge from pandemics, we need an honest conversation about how to strike a balance between maintaining necessary steps to mitigate ongoing risk and supporting the resumption of normal life. This means working to protect the vulnerable as long as needed while differentiating between their needs and those of the general population.

62

COVID-19 AND THE OFFICE

Prior to the pandemic, an estimated 95 million workers had jobs that required physical attendance and interaction with others. Before COVID-19 vaccines were available, tens of millions of Americans continued to head off to their jobs as delivery drivers, grocery store staff, and other kinds of frontline workers, unprotected amid the pandemic's dangers. When COVID-19 struck, this status quo faced deep disruption. Some work, notably in the travel and hospitality industries, simply disappeared. Forty percent of American workers, or 63 million, were employed in occupations that potentially could be performed remotely, an option in large part driven by education level and reflecting a racial disparity: Only 16.2 percent of Hispanic workers and 19.7 percent of Black workers could telework.

Yet as COVID-19 closed large segments of the economy, media coverage focused on those privileged office jobs that were undergoing a transformational experiment in the possibility of remote work. Suddenly, the stigma of working remotely—a practice once seen as unproductive—was reduced. This raised the question: Would these changes to offices last?

The idea of office work originally emerged in an industrial context. The factory was the paradigm for nine-to-five indoor work.

The Turning Point. Michael D. Stein and Sandro Galea, Oxford University Press.
© Oxford University Press 2024. DOI: 10.1093/oso/9780197749685.003.0062

The office became another kind of factory floor, giving employers the possibility of surveillance, of ensuring that workers were working. In office settings, managers were able to assign and track work efficiently. For employers, the office became a place to onboard new workers, create teams, and oversee shirkers. For the employee, the office became a site for collaboration as well as structured work, a place to make friends and have a social life, a destination apart from the domestic sphere.

White collar workplaces have never functioned like the manufacturing, construction, food service, and health care sectors where federal agencies such as the Occupational Safety and Health Administration set worker protection rules. When telework was not possible during the pandemic, fatal hazard entered the office world, as did possible liability issues. Thus, the new workplace had a temperature checking station, an isolation room, a handwashing area, and lockers for outside clothes and shoes. There were touchless entry doors, coffee machines, water coolers, and utensil drawers. Industry standards around health changed in many places. Yet the risk-mitigation measure that works best to limit transmission and keep people safe indoors should have long predated COVID-19—this is, the installation of proper air filtration systems. By 2021, positive COVID-19 cases did not automatically derail reopening plans. Decisions often came down to perception of risk and managing high levels of anxiety. It was mostly collective fear that pushed employees away from the office and supervisors to close shop, rather than government-imposed lockdowns leading to the closure of businesses.

Whereas in the first year of the pandemic, one-third of the labor force worked remotely, a year later less than half that number remained remote. Digital technology was not a substitute for human connection. Yet as the memory of the pandemic recedes, employers and employees alike will likely continue to ask, Is the office worth its price?

63

A COVID-19
POVERTY SURPRISE

The U.S. Congress provided three rounds of stimulus checks to American workers starting in March 2020, the first month that COVID-19 shuttered many parts of the economy. Unemployment insurance payments began to reach workers never previously eligible. Supplemental Nutrition Assistance Program (SNAP) food vouchers doubled. An emergency rental aid program was created that suddenly matched the entire annual budget of the Department of Housing and Urban Development. The social safety net finally got some bounce to it. By the start of 2021, poverty in America had plummeted to an all-time low. Indeed, lost in the story of COVID-19 was the story of how the United States showed that it could, and did, curb poverty.

Nearly 60 percent of Americans will experience poverty (currently defined as a family of four with an annual income less than $30,000) before they turn age 75 years. Poverty at this level is intergenerational—income class mobility is limited. Children born poor tend to stay that way. Poverty, of course, is the most significant determinant of children and young people's health. The pervasive influence of poverty was amply illustrated by the

The Turning Point. Michael D. Stein and Sandro Galea, Oxford University Press.
© Oxford University Press 2024. DOI: 10.1093/oso/9780197749685.003.0063

observation that the poorest among us suffered the worst health consequences of COVID-19.

It took \$4.5 trillion allocated to COVID-19 relief—a figure that exceeded the entire federal budget in 2019—to make the hardships of 2020 more tolerable for many of the most vulnerable. Even as millions lost jobs, at the start of 2021, 20 million fewer Americans were in poverty—a remarkable and historically unprecedented improvement. With Congressional bills focused on short-term recovery, the decline in poverty was proportionally greatest among children. But poverty declined among Black, Latinos, and Whites, across every age group, and in every state. Contemporaneously, hunger did not rise in 2020.

What is the long-term benefit of this historic change in priorities in this expansion of the welfare state? It will depend on which parts last. SNAP, for example, modified its assumptions about what constitutes an adequate diet, which determines the size of monthly benefits; this re-examination of healthy eating was accelerated by COVID-19, and this investment will last for decades. But whether changes in guaranteed income for families with children, a 2020 innovation, become part of the new rigging of the safety net remains to be seen. The National Academies of Sciences, Engineering, and Medicine suggests that unconditional cash aid leads poor children to higher earnings as adults, fewer arrests, and better health. The question, then, is whether this will become part of the permanent fabric of supports in this country.

COVID-19 obliged us to test an abundance of new national policies, from travel restrictions to vaccine mandates, from U.S.

Food and Drug Administration regulation to industry-specific economic shutdowns. Among the most profound tests had been whether we could make a dent in poverty at a moment of desperate need. We saw that we can. It is now clear that our ability to address, or not address, poverty more permanently is a political choice.

64

IS IT OVER YET?

Throughout the United States, over the course of a few months, there were approximately 21 million symptomatic cases, 290,000 hospitalizations, and 37,000 deaths. More than 25,000 of the deaths were in the 65+ years age group.

It seems likely that this type of case and death count recitation is familiar to the reader, seen through the lens of COVID-19, when we assiduously documented cases and deaths for the greater part of two years. But these were not COVID-19 numbers. They were cases, and deaths, from flu during the 2010–2011 influenza season, one of the worst seasons in the past decade. This begs the question: How many of us were aware of the daily case and death count during that flu season? And, perhaps more important, would we have behaved differently as a society if we had been keeping track of cases and deaths the way we did during COVID-19?

In some ways, COVID-19 case and death counting took on an uncomfortably familiar role, with tallies being reported in all media in much the same way as, for example, the weather, which is also reported daily. But what impact did this abundance of reporting have on how we thought about the pandemic?

Testing for COVID-19 was one of the issues that became politicized during the Trump presidency, perhaps most

The Turning Point, Michael D. Stein and Sandro Galea, Oxford University Press.
© Oxford University Press 2024. DOI: 10.1093/oso/9780197749685.003.0064

dramatically because it seemed that the president was suggesting that we should not test for COVID-19 so as not to raise alarm about the scale of the pandemic. That approach, in June 2020, would have been disastrous. Testing and counting cases of a disease are the cornerstones of epidemiology and allow us to document the scope and spread of contagion. Testing allows new variants to be identified. It is a measurement that allowed us to better understand the groups that were most at risk for COVID-19, and it is routine testing that allowed universities to stay safe, through intensive efforts to screen for early cases and prevent them from becoming clusters leading to outbreaks.

But, as the pandemic ebbed and flowed, as vaccination reached more than 70 percent of the population, the question arose: Did the omnipresence of case counts give us an impression of risk that was at odds with real risk? Daily COVID-19 case statistics above the fold in our newspapers suggested these numbers were urgent news. But this overexposure may have been read as a recommendation to continue isolation unnecessarily and made us unfortunately reluctant to mingle. That many aspects of this approach to the pandemic continued for more than three years after the virus first emerged reflects our inability to adapt to an evolving public health challenge. We need to do better. COVID-19 will not be the last such challenge we face, and the rigidity of our approach will not serve us well in the future. This suggests the importance of conversations about when it is appropriate to continue counting cases—of any disease—and when it might be counterproductive to do so.

65

NOW WHAT?

We conclude this book with a simple question: What comes next?

When the public health emergency was declared at an end in the United States on May 11, 2023, after three years, more than 1.1 million Americans, and more than 6 million people worldwide, had died of COVID-19. More than 750 million people were infected throughout the world. COVID-19 is now ubiquitous, and we live in a world in which nearly every young child has acquired a measure of immunity against a virus unknown only a few years ago. The health effects of long COVID will likely affect millions worldwide. And it is clear that the health consequences of the economic and social upheaval due to COVID-19—mental illness, drug overdose, higher death rates from heart disease—will stay with us for years to come. An unprecedented global effort to vaccinate as many people as possible delivered successes—notably a historic rapid development of safe and effective vaccines delivered to billions of people in record time—and many failures—notably the patchy delivery of vaccines to low-income countries and the uneven distribution of vaccines within high-income countries.

Now what?

The Turning Point. Michael D. Stein and Sandro Galea. Oxford University Press.
© Oxford University Press 2024. DOI: 10.1093/oso/9780197749685.003.0065

It would be a fool's errand to try to predict the future. If nothing else, the COVID-19 years were characterized by a series of misestimations of the course of the disease, by hope that the pandemic would be behind us soon dashed by viral resurgence or variants, with mounting numbers of new infections. The pandemic taught us that it is a complex mix of viral dynamics and human behavior that determines the burden of the disease and that efforts at predicting what is around the corner are, at best, informed guesses.

But what we do know is that the moment has much to teach us and that if we learn the right lessons we will be better prepared to deal with the next pandemic.

One lesson has been that we should avoid the temptation to think that there is a simple solution to our predicament. Complex systems resist simple answers.

Wisdom lies in having the humility to recognize that future success is not only about getting to better vaccines faster but also in ensuring that we have a healthier world that is resistant to new pandemics. Much of what we got wrong during COVID-19 was due to an inattention to health that long predated COVID-19.

As we reflect on the ideas that emerged as the pandemic evolved, we see how much we still have to learn. We look forward to continuing this reflection as the public conversation evolves.

BIBLIOGRAPHY

Section 1. Lessons

1. From Theory to Practice

1. COVID-19 vaccinations: County and state tracker. (2020). *The New York Times*. Retrieved January 7, 2022, from https://www.nytimes.com/interactive/2020/us/covid-19-vaccine-doses.html
2. Goldman, P., & Saphora, S. (2021, January 3). *Paralyzed by COVID-19, Israel bids to be first country to vaccinate its way to safety*. NBC News. Retrieved January 7, 2022, from https://www.nbcnews.com/news/world/paralyzed-COVID-19-israel-bids-be-first-country-vaccinate-its-n1252682
3. Lupkin, S. (2020, December 23). *U.S. government to buy additional 100 million doses of Pfizer COVID-19 vaccine*. NPR. Retrieved January 7, 2022, from https://www.npr.org/2020/12/23/949751699/u-s-government-to-buy-additional-100-million-doses-of-pfizer-COVID-19-vaccine
4. McElhinny, B. (2020, December 21). *West Virginia may complete nursing home vaccinations even sooner than expected*. MetroNews. Retrieved January 7, 2022, from https://wvmetronews.com/2020/12/21/west-virginia-may-complete-nursing-home-vaccinations-even-sooner-than-expected

3. The Irreplaceable Public Sector

1. Weinberg, A. (2021, April 28). Joe Biden rolls out the sleepy new deal. *Mother Jones*. Retrieved January 7, 2022, from https://www.motherjones.com/mojo-wire/2021/04/joe-biden-rolls-out-the-sleepy-new-deal
2. *How "government" became a dirty word*. (2012, September 1). NPR. Retrieved January 7, 2022, from https://www.npr.org/2012/09/01/160438753/how-government-became-a-dirty-word
3. United States COVID—Coronavirus statistics. (n.d.). Worldometer. Retrieved January 7, 2022, from https://www.worldometers.info/coronavirus/country/us

4. Holding Our Breath

1. Chu, H., Englund, J., Starita, L., Famulare, M., Brandstetter, E., Nickerson, D., Rieder, M., Adler, A., Lacombe, K., Kim, A., Graham, C., Logue, J., Wolf, C., Heimonen, J., McCulloch, D., Han, P., Sibley, T., Lee, J., Ilcisin, M., . . . Bedford, T.; for the Seattle Flu Study Investigators. (2020, May 1). Early detection of COVID-19 through a citywide pandemic surveillance platform. *New England Journal of Medicine, 383*, 185–187. https://www.nejm.org/doi/full/10.1056/NEJMc2008646

2. Biofire Diagnostics. (n.d.). *Respiratory pathogen trends.* Retrieved January 7, 2022, from https://syndromictrends.com

3. Centers for Disease Control and Prevention. (2021). *RSV national trends.* Retrieved January 7, 2022, from https://www.cdc.gov/surveillance/nrevss/rsv/natl-trend.html

4. Centers for Disease Control and Prevention. (2021). *Influenza vaccinations administered in pharmacies and physician medical offices, adults, United States.* Retrieved January 7, 2022, from https://www.cdc.gov/flu/fluvaxview/dashboard/vaccination-administered.html?web=1&wdLOR=c7046EB18-6B17-8D47-A7D3-6A2E0FEBA4E8

5. Walker, A. S. (2022, December 16). *Just how bad is the "tripledemic"? The New York Times.* Retrieved January 13, 2023, from https://www.nytimes.com/interactive/2022/12/16/us/covid-flu-rsv-tripledemic-data.html

6. Kekatos, M. (2022, December 16). *After fears of "tripledemic," RSV on the downturn as flu and COVID pick up.* ABC News. Retrieved January 13, 2023, from https://abcnews.go.com/Health/after-fears-tripledemic-rsv-downturn-flu-covid-pick/story?id=95418846

5. The Challenge of Addressing Multiple Crises

1. *Timeline: The events leading up to Russia's invasion of Ukraine.* (2022, March 1). Reuters. Retrieved February 1, 2023, from https://www.reuters.com/world/europe/events-leading-up-russias-invasion-ukraine-2022-02-28

2. Myre, G. (2022, updated October 4). *How likely is a Russian nuclear strike in Ukraine?* NPR. Retrieved February 1, 2023, from https://www.npr.org/2022/10/04/1126680868/putin-raises-the-specter-of-using-nuclear-weapons-in-his-war-with-ukraine

3. Thomas, M. B. (2020, November 24). *Epidemics on the move: Climate change and infectious disease. PLoS Biology, 18*(11), e3001013. https://journals.plos.org/plosbiology/article?id=10.1371/journal.pbio.3001013

4. Hultman, N. (2018, October 16). *We're almost out of time: The alarming IPCC climate report and what to do next.* Brookings. Retrieved January 7, 2022, from https://www.brookings.edu/opinions/were-almost-out-of-time-the-alarming-ipcc-climate-report-and-what-to-do-next

5. Morrison, J. (2019, August 5). *Who will pay for the huge costs of holding back rising seas? Yale Environment 360.* Retrieved January 7, 2022, from https://e360.yale.edu/features/who-will-pay-for-the-huge-costs-of-holding-back-rising-seas

6. Le Quéré, C., Jackson, R. B., Jones, M. W., Smith, A., Abernethy, S., Andrew, R., De-Gol, A., Willis, D., Shan, Y., Canadell, J., Friedlingstein, P., Creutzig, F., & Peters, G. (2020). Temporary reduction in daily global CO_2 emissions during the COVID-19 forced confinement. *Nature Climate Change, 10,* 647–653.

7. Marcacci, S. (2020, June 9). Plunging renewable energy prices mean U.S. can hit 90% clean electricity by 2035—at no extra cost. *Forbes.* Retrieved January 7, 2022, from https://www.forbes.com/sites/energyinnovation/2020/06/09/plunging-renewable-energy-prices-mean-us-can-hit-90-clean-electricity-by-2035at-no-extra-cost/?sh=6b5626c22f9b

6. The Invisible Mental Health Burdens of a Pandemic

1. Riehm, K. E., Holingue, C., Smail, E. J., Kapteyn, A., Bennett, D., Thrul, J., Kreuter, F., McGinty, E. E., Kalb, L. G., Veldhuis, C. B., Johnson, R. M., Fallin, M. D., & Stuart, E. A. (2021). Trajectories of mental distress among U.S. adults during the COVID-19 pandemic. *Annals of Behavioral Medicine, 55*(2), 93–102.

2. COVID-19 Mental Disorders Collaborators. (2021). Global prevalence and burden of depressive and anxiety disorders in 204 countries and territories in 2020 due to the COVID-19 pandemic. *Lancet, 398*(10312), 1700–1712.

3. Goldmann, E., & Galea, S. (2013). Mental health consequences of disasters. *Annual Review of Public Health, 35,* 169–183.

4. Bridgland, V. M., Moeck, E. K., Green, D. M., Swain, T. L., Nayda, D. M., Matson, L. A., Hutchison, N. P., & Takarangi, M. K. T. (2021). Why the COVID-19 pandemic is a traumatic stressor. *PLoS One, 16*(1), e240146.

5. Ettman, C. K., Abdalla, S. M., Cohen, G. H., Sampson, L., Vivier, P. M., & Galea, S. (2020). Prevalence of depression symptoms in US adults before and during the COVID-19 pandemic. *JAMA, 3*(9), e2019686.

6. Jia, H., Guerin, R. J., Barile, J. P., Okun, A. H., McKnight-Eily, L., Blumberg, S. J., Njai, R., & Thompson, W. W. (2021). National and state trends in anxiety and depression severity scores among adults during the COVID-19 pandemic—United States, 2020–2021. *MMWR: Morbidity and Mortality Weekly Report, 70*(40), 1427–1432.

7. Ettman, C. K., Cohen, G. H., Abdalla, S. M., Sampson, L., Trinquart, L., Castrucci, B. C., Bork, R. H., Clark, M. A., Wilson, I., Vivier, P. M., & Galea, S. (2021). Persistent depressive symptoms during COVID-19: A national, population-representative, longitudinal study of U.S. adults. *Lancet Regional Health Americas, 5,* 100091.

8. Fatollahi, J. J., Bentley, S., Doran, N., & Brody, A. L. (2021). Changes in tobacco use patterns among veterans in San Diego during the recent peak of the COVID-19 pandemic. *International Journal of Environmental Research and Public Health, 18*(22), 11923.

9. Killgore, W. D., Cloonan, S. A., Taylor, E. C., Lucas, D. A., & Dailey, N. S. (2021). Morning drinking during COVID-19 lockdowns. *Psychiatry Research, 307,* 114320.

10. Kamp, J., & Wernau, J. (2021, November 17). Drug overdose deaths, fueled by fentanyl, hit record high in U.S. *The Wall Street Journal.* Retrieved January 7, 2022, from https://www.wsj.com/articles/drug-overdose-deaths-fueled-by-fentanyl-hit-record-high-in-u-s-11637161200?mod=article_inline

11. Bryant, M. K., Aubry, S., Schiro, S., Raff, L., Perez, A. J., Reid, T., & Maine, R. G. (2021). Causes of death following discharge after trauma in North Carolina. *Journal of Trauma and Acute Care Surgery, 92*(2), 371–379.

12. Institute for Crime & Justice Policy Research. (2021, January 12). *World prison population list.* Retrieved January 7, 2022, from https://www.prisonstudies.org/sites/default/files/resources/downloads/world_prison_population_list_13th_edition.pdf

7. Pandemics and Prisons

1. Drucker, E. (2013). *The plague of prisons: The epidemiology of mass incarceration in America.* New Press.

2. New York Association of Psychiatric Rehabilitation Services. (2020, May 26). *New report shows high link between suicide and solitary confinement, Advocates demand that Governor Cuomo, state legislators act now!* Retrieved January 7, 2022, from https://www.nyaprs.org/e-news-bulletins/2020/5/26/new-rep

ort-shows-high-link-between-suicide-and-solitary-confinement-advoca
tes-demand-that-governor-cuomo-state-legislators-act-now

3. Katz, B. (2019, March 6). Nearly half of Americans have a close family
member who has been incarcerated. *Smithsonian Magazine.* Retrieved
January 7, 2022, from https://www.smithsonianmag.com/smart-news/
nearly-half-americans-have-close-family-member-who-has-been-
incarcerated-180971645

4. Prison Policy Initiative. (2021). *The most significant criminal justice
policy changes from the COVID-19 pandemic.* Retrieved January 7, 2022,
from:https://www.prisonpolicy.org/virus/virusresponse.html

5. National Commission on COVID-19 and Criminal Justice. (2020,
September 2). *Impact report: COVID-19 and prisons.* Retrieved January 7,
2022, from https://covid19.counciloncj.org/2020/09/02/COVID-19-and-
prisons

6. The COVID Prison Project. (n.d.). Retrieved January 7, 2022, from
https://covidprisonproject.com

7. Ella Baker Center. (2015, September). *Who pays? The true cost of incarceration on families.* Retrieved January 16, 2022, from https://ellabakercenter.
org/who-pays-the-true-cost-of-incarceration-on-families

8. The Necessity of Speaking with Care

1. *The Brothers Karamazov study guide.* (n.d.). SparkNotes. Retrieved
February 1, 2023, from https://www.sparknotes.com/lit/brothersk/
character/ivan

2. Zizek, S. (2012, April 16). *If there is a God, then anything is permitted.* ABC
News (Australian Broadcasting Corporation). Retrieved February 1,
2023, from https://www.abc.net.au/religion/if-there-is-a-god-then-
anything-is-permitted/10100616

3. Su, Z., Cheshmehzangi, A., McDonnell, D., Ahmad, J., Segalo, S., Xiang,
Y. T., & da Veiga, C. P. (2022). The advantages of the zero-COVID-19
strategy. *International Journal of Environmental Research and Public Health,*
19(14), 8767.

4. Yiu, K. (2022, November 27). *How a deadly apartment fire fueled anti-zero-
COVID protests across China: Analysis.* ABC News. Retrieved February 1,
2023, from https://abcnews.go.com/International/deadly-apartment-
fire-fueled-anti-zero-covid-protests/story?id=94045207

5. Human Rights Watch. (n.d.). *Mass surveillance in China.* Retrieved
February 1, 2023, from https://www.hrw.org/tag/mass-surveilla
nce-china

6. *Who are the Uyghurs and why is China being accused of genocide?* (2022, May 24). BBC News. Retrieved February 1, 2023, from https://www.bbc.com/news/world-asia-china-22278037

9. Health Behavior

1. Jay, J., Bor, J., Nsoesie, E. O., Lipson, S. K., Jones, D. K., Galea, S., & Raifman, J. (2020). Neighbourhood income and physical distancing during the COVID-19 pandemic in the United States. *Nature Human Behaviour, 4*(12), 1294–1302.
2. Dores, A. R., Carvalho, I. P., Burkauskas, J., Simonato, P., De Luca, I., Mooney, R., Ioannidis, K., Gomez-Martinez, M. A., Demetrovics, Z., Abel, K. E., Szabo, A., Fujiwara, H., Shibata, M., Melero Ventola, A. R., Arroyo-Anllo, E. M., Santos-Labrador, R. M., Griskova-Bulanova, I., Pranckeviciene, A., Kobayashi, K., . . . Corazza, O. (2021). Exercise and use of enhancement drugs at the time of the COVID-19 pandemic: A multicultural study on coping strategies during self-isolation and related risks. *Frontiers in Psychiatry, 12,* 648501.
3. Holland, K. M., Jones, C., Vivolo-Kantor, A. M., Idaikkadar, N., Zwald, M., Hoots, B., Yard, E., D'Inverno, A., Swedo, E., Chen, M. S., Petrosky, E., Board, A., Martinez, P., Stone, D. M., Law, R., Coletta, M. A., Adjemian, J., Thomas, C., Puddy, R. W., . . . Houry, D. (2021). Trends in US emergency department visits for mental health, overdose, and violence outcomes before and during the COVID-19 pandemic. *JAMA Psychiatry, 78*(4), 372–379.
4. Hollands, G. J., French, D. P., Griffin, S. J., Provost, A. T., Sutton, S., King, S., & Marteau, T. M. (2016). The impact of communicating genetic risks of disease on risk-reducing health behaviour: Systematic review with meta-analysis. *BMJ, 15*(352), i1102.
5. Shreffler, J., Shoff, H., Thomas, J. J., & Huecker, M. (2021). Brief report: The impact of COVID-19 on emergency department overdose diagnoses and county overdose deaths. *American Journal of Addiction, 30*(4), 330–333.
6. Fenichel, E. P., Castillo-Chavez, C., Ceddia, M. G., Chowell, G., Gonzalez Parra, P. A., Hickling, G. J., Holloway, G., Horan, R., Morin, B., Perrings, C., Springborn, M., Velazquez, L., & Villalobos, C. (2011). Adaptive human behavior in epidemiological models. *Proceedings of the National Academy of Sciences of the USA, 108*(15), 6306–6311.

11. Does Today Matter More Than Tomorrow?

1. *Time (temporal) discounting.* (n.d.). Behavioral Economics. Retrieved January 7, 2022, from https://www.behavioraleconomics.com/resour ces/mini-encyclopedia-of-be/time-temporal-discounting
2. Woolf, S. H., Chapman, D. A., Sabo, R. T., Weinberger, D. M., Hill, L., & Taylor, D. D. (2020). Excess deaths from COVID-19 and other causes, March–July 2020. *JAMA, 324*(15), 1562–1564.
3. Panchal, N., Kamal, R., Cox, C., & Garfield, R. (2021, February 10). *The implications of COVID-19 for mental health and substance use.* KFF. Retrieved January 7, 2022, from https://www.kff.org/coronavirus-COVID-19/ issue-brief/the-implications-of-COVID-19-for-mental-health-and-substance-use
4. Ettman, C. K., Abdalla, S. M., Cohen, G. H., Sampson, L., Vivier, P. M., & Galea, S. (2020). Prevalence of depression symptoms in US adults before and during the COVID-19 pandemic. *JAMA Network Open, 3*(9), e20196861–12.
5. MindTools Content Team. (n.d.). *Eisenhower's urgent/important principle.* MindTools. Retrieved January 7, 2022, from https://www.mindtools. com/pages/article/newHTE_91.htm

12. Telling Different Stories with the Same Data

1. *Tokyo 2020 Olympics: Final medal table.* (2021, August 6). *The Guardian.* Retrieved January 7, 2022, from https://www.theguardian.com/sport/ ng-interactive/2021/aug/06/tokyo-2020-olympics-full-medal-table
2. Dure, B. (2021, August 7). Team USA top the Olympic medal table. Or is it China? Or . . . San Marino? *The Guardian.* Retrieved January 7, 2022, from https://www.theguardian.com/sport/2021/aug/07/olympics-medal-table-formats-best-countries
3. Ortaliza, J., Ramirez, G., Satheeskumar, V., & Amin, K. (2021, September 8). *How does U.S. life expectancy compare to other countries?* Peterson–KFF Health System Tracker. Retrieved January 7, 2022, from https://www. healthsystemtracker.org/chart-collection/u-s-life-expectancy-comp are-countries/#item-le_life-expectancy-in-years-at-given-age-2017_ dec-2019-update
4. Galea, S. (2016, August 25). The case for public health, In 18 charts. *HuffPost.* Retrieved January 7, 2022, from https://www.huffpost.com/ entry/the-case-for-public-healt_b_11699182

5. National Research Council, Institute of Medicine; Woolf, S. H., & Aron, L. (Eds.). (2013). *U.S. health in international perspective: Shorter lives, poorer health*. National Academies Press.

6. Stein, M., & Galea, S. (2021, June 10). Defining our goalposts. *Public Health Post*. Retrieved January 7, 2022, from https://www.publichealthp ost.org/the-turning-point/defining-our-goalposts

7. Stein, M., & Galea, S. (2021, February 5). Achieving health equity, efficiently. *Public Health Post*. Retrieved January 7, 2022, from https://www.publichealthpost.org/the-turning-point/achieving-health-equity-effi ciently

8. Wagner, M., Macaya, M., Mahtani, M., & Rocha, V. (2021, August 2). *August 2, 2021 US coronavirus news*. CNN. Retrieved January 7, 2022, from https://www.cnn.com/us/live-news/coronavirus-pandemic-vaccine-updates-08-02-21/h_4258aa07cbf2206435b5f84328ddab33

9. Owens, C. (2021, August 4). *America's pandemic pessimism returns*. Axios. Retrieved January 7, 2022, from https://www.axios.com/america-pandemic-polling-coronavirus-pessimism-8c1584dd-2aab-446b-825c-ab2aa8454c9e.html

10. Galea, S. (2021, July 17). *A playbook for balancing the moral and empirical case for health*. Substack. Retrieved January 7, 2022, from https://sandroga lea.substack.com/p/a-playbook-for-balancing-the-moral

13. How Our Expectations Shape Our Perceptions of Reality

1. Rich, M. (2021, August 5). Second best in the world, but still saying sorry. *The New York Times*. Retrieved January 7, 2022, from https://www.nytimes.com/2021/08/05/world/asia/japan-olympics-apology.html

2. Miller, Z. (2021, June 15). *"A summer of freedom": Vaccine gives new meaning to July 4th*. Associated Press. Retrieved January 7, 2022, from https://apnews.com/article/government-and-politics-joe-biden-lifestyle-coro navirus-pandemic-health-f97e0316c51d2d8362a17d149daedb14

3. Owens, C. (2021, August 4). *America's pandemic pessimism returns*. Axios. Retrieved January 7, 2022, from https://www.axios.com/america-pandemic-polling-coronavirus-pessimism-8c1584dd-2aab-446b-825c-ab2aa8454c9e.html

4. Chiwaya, N. (2021, July 28). *Map: Covid cases are rising in the states with low vaccination rates*. NBC News. Retrieved January 7, 2022, from https://www.nbcnews.com/news/us-news/map-covid-cases-are-rising-sta tes-low-vaccination-rates-n1275322

5. Centers for Disease Control and Prevention. (n.d.). *Science brief: COVID-19 vaccines and vaccination*. Retrieved January 7, 2022, from https://www.cdc. gov/coronavirus/2019-ncov/science/science-briefs/fully-vaccinated-people.html

14. Can Contact Tracing Work Here?

1. Beaubien, J. (2020, March 1). *Hong Kong has contained coronavirus so far—but at a significant cost*. NPR KQED. Retrieved January 7, 2022, from https:// www.npr.org/sections/goatsandsoda/2020/03/01/810392094/hong-kong-has-contained-coronavirus-so-far-but-at-a-significant-cost

2. Beaubien, J. (2020, March 12). *Singapore wins praise for its COVID-19 strategy. The U.S. does not*. NPR KQED. Retrieved January 7, 2022, from https:// www.npr.org/sections/goatsandsoda/2020/03/12/814522489/singap ore-wins-praise-for-its-COVID-19-strategy-the-u-s-does-not

3. Stein, M., & Galea, S. (2021, March 11). Next time, testing first. *Public Health Post*. Retrieved January 7, 2022, from https://www.publichealthpost.org/ the-turning-point/next-time-testing-first

4. Ordoñez, F. (2020, April 27). *Ex-officials call for $46 billion for tracing, isolating in next coronavirus package*. NPR KQED. Retrieved January 7, 2022, from https://www.npr.org/2020/04/27/845165404/ex-officials-call-for-46-billion-for-tracing-isolating-in-next-coronavirus-packa

5. Lash, R. R., Moonan, P. K., Byers, B. L., Bonacci, R., Bonner, K., Donahue, M., Donovan, C., Grome, H., Janssen, J., Magleby, R., McLaughlin, H., Miller, J., Pratt, C., Steinberg, J., Varela, K., Anschuetz, G., Cieslak, P., Fialkowsik, V., & Goddard, C.; COVID-19 Contact Tracing Assessment Team. (2021). COVID-19 case investigation and contact tracing in the US, 2020. *JAMA Network Open, 4*(6), e2115850.

15. Prescription Against Worry

1. U.S. Food and Drug Administration. (2021, December 23). *Coronavirus (COVID-19) update: FDA authorizes additional oral antiviral for treatment of COVID-19 in certain adults*. . Retrieved January 7, 2022, from https://www. fda.gov/news-events/press-announcements/coronavirus-COVID-19-upd ate-fda-authorizes-additional-oral-antiviral-treatment-COVID-19-certain

2. Centers for Disease Control and Prevention. (n.d.). *Overview of testing for SARS-CoV-2, the virus that causes COVID-19*. Retrieved January 7, 2022, from https://www.cdc.gov/coronavirus/2019-ncov/hcp/testing-overview.html

3. Yang, J. (2021, November 17). *Number of people without health insurance in the United States from 1997 to June 2021.* Statista. Retrieved January 7, 2022, from https://www.statista.com/statistics/200955/americans-without-health-insurance

Section 2. Story

16. Political Decisions and Science

1. Finucane, M., Huddle, R., & Andersen, T. (2021, January 22). After Baker relaxes some pandemic restrictions, epidemiologists urge caution. *The Boston Globe.* Retrieved January 7, 2022, from https://www.bostonglobe.com/2021/01/23/nation/after-baker-relaxes-some-pandemic-restrictions-epidemiologists-urge-caution
2. Green, E. (2021, January 24). Surge of student suicides pushes Las Vegas schools to reopen. *The New York Times.* Retrieved January 7, 2022, from https://www.nytimes.com/2021/01/24/us/politics/student-suicides-nevada-coronavirus.html
3. Centers for Disease Control and Prevention. (2020, July 24). *Transcript for CDC telebriefing on new resources and tools to support opening schools.* Retrieved January 7, 2022, from https://www.cdc.gov/media/releases/2020/t0724-new-resources-tools-schools.html

19. Defining Our Goalposts

1. Finelli, L., Gupta, V., Petigara, T., Yu, K., Bauer, K. A., & Puzniak, L. A. (2021). Mortality among US patients hospitalized with SARS-CoV-2 infection in 2020. *JAMA Network Open, 4*(4), e216556.
2. Thompson, A. E., Ranard, B. L., Wei, Y., & Jelic, S. (2020). Prone positioning in awake, nonintubated patients with COVID-19 hypoxemic respiratory failure. *JAMA Internal Medicine, 180*(11), 1537–1539.
3. Centers for Disease Control and Prevention. (n.d.). *COVID data tracker weekly review.* Retrieved January 7, 2022, from https://www.cdc.gov/coronavirus/2019-ncov/covid-data/covidview/index.html

20. The Limits of Our Science

1. Saag, M. S. (2020). Misguided use of hydroxychloroquine for COVID-19: The infusion of politics into science. *JAMA, 324*(21), 2161–2162.

2. Biden, J. (2020, May 21). *Tweet*. Twitter. Retrieved January 8, 2022, from https://twitter.com/joebiden/status/1263509860395610113?lang=en

3. Maani, N., & Galea, S. (2021, February 2). What science can and cannot do in a time of pandemic. *Scientific American*. Retrieved January 8, 2022, from https://www.scientificamerican.com/article/what-science-can-and-cannot-do-in-a-time-of-pandemic

4. Ries, J. (2021, February 11). *Kids are half as likely to get COVID-19 as adults: Here's what we know*. Healthline. Retrieved January 8, 2022, from https://www.healthline.com/health-news/kids-are-half-as-likely-get-COVID-19-as-adults-heres-what-we-know

5. Lewis, D. (2020) Why schools probably aren't COVID hotspots. *Nature*, 587(7832), Article 17.

6. Jaschik, S. (2012, October 24). Moving further to the left. *Inside Higher Ed*. Retrieved January 8, 2022, from https://www.insidehighered.com/news/2012/10/24/survey-finds-professors-already-liberal-have-moved-further-left

7. Sakal, V. (2021, January 19). *An inaugural inflection point: Ushering in a new era of marketing amid a polarized public*. Morning Consult. Retrieved January 8, 2022, from https://morningconsult.com/2021/01/19/an-inaugural-inflection-point-ushering-in-a-new-era-of-marketing-amid-a-polarized-public

21. The National Character

1. Ravelo, J. L., & Jerving, S. (n.d.). *COVID-19 in 2020—A timeline of the coronavirus outbreak*. Devex. Retrieved January 8, 2022, from https://www.devex.com/news/COVID-19-in-2020-a-timeline-of-the-coronavirus-outbreak-99634

2. Ramzy, A., & Dong, J. (2021, October 26). China locks down a northwestern city to subdue a small outbreak. *The New York Times*. Retrieved January 8, 2022, from https://www.nytimes.com/2021/10/26/world/asia/covid-china-lanzhou-lockdown.html

3. Shuren, J., & Stenzel, T. (2021, May 25). South Korea's implementation of a COVID-19 national testing strategy. *Health Affairs*. Retrieved January 8, 2022, from https://www.healthaffairs.org/do/10.1377/forefront.20210521.255232/full

4. Dyer, P. (2021, June 15). *Policy and institutional responses to COVID-19: South Korea*. Brookings. Retrieved January 8, 2022, from https://

www.brookings.edu/research/policy-and-institutional-respon ses-to-COVID-19-south-korea

5. Maani, N., & Galea, S. (2020). COVID-19 and underinvestment in the public health infrastructure of the United States. *Milbank Quarterly, 98*(2), 250–259.

6. Bradsher, K. (2022, December 9). Beijing braces for Covid surge after China lifts pandemic curbs. *The New York Times*. Retrieved January 14, 2023, from https://www.nytimes.com/2022/12/09/world/asia/beijing-china-covid.html

7. McDonald, J. (2022, December 7). *China eases anti-COVID measures following protests*. Associated Press. Retrieved February 1, 2023, from https://apnews.com/article/health-business-china-covid-economy-e5559f606 2cf052a71ad6ba1ceece693

22. The Right to Bear News

1. Sacerdote, B., Sehgal, R., & Cook, M. (2020, November). *Why is all COVID-19 news bad news?* Retrieved January 8, 2022, from https://cpb-us-e1.wpmucdn.com/sites.dartmouth.edu/dist/4/2318/files/2021/03/Why-Is-All-Covid-News-Bad-News-3_22_21.pdf

2. Leonhardt, D. (2021, March 24). Covid coverage by the U.S. national media is an outlier, a study finds. *The New York Times*. Retrieved January 8, 2022, from https://www.nytimes.com/2021/03/24/world/covid-coverage-by-the-us-national-media-is-an-outlier-a-study-finds.html

3. Centers for Disease Control and Prevention. (2021, July 14). *Drug overdose deaths in the U.S. up 30% in 2020*. Retrieved January 8, 2022, from https://www.cdc.gov/nchs/pressroom/nchs_press_releases/2021/20210 714.htm

4. Ettman, C. K., Cohen, G. H., Abdalla, S. M., Sampson, L., Trinquart, L., Castrucci, B. C., Bork, R. H., Clark, M. A., Wilson, I., Vivier, P. M., & Galea, S. (2021). Persistent depressive symptoms during COVID-19: A national, population-representative, longitudinal study of U.S. adults. *Lancet Regional Health Americas, 5,* 100091.

23. The Story of COVID-19

1. Cinelli, M., Quattrociocchi, W., Galeazzi, A., Valensise, C. M., Brugnoli, E., Schmidt, A. L., Zola, P., Zollo, F., & Scala, A. (2020). The COVID-19 social media infodemic. *Scientific Reports, 10,* 16598.

2. Centers for Disease Control and Prevention. (n.d.). *Understanding How COVID-19 Vaccines Work*. Retrieved January 8, 2022, from https://www.cdc.gov/coronavirus/2019-ncov/vaccines/different-vaccines/how-they-work.html

3. Gould, E., & Wilson, V. (2020, June 1). *Black workers face two of the most lethal preexisting conditions for coronavirus—racism and economic inequality*. Economic Policy Institute. Retrieved January 8, 2022, from https://www.epi.org/publication/black-workers-covid

4. Centers for Disease Control and Prevention. (n.d.). *African American health*. Retrieved January 8, 2022, from https://www.cdc.gov/vitalsigns/aahealth/index.html

5. Falk, G., Romero, P. D., Nicchitta, I. A., & Nyhof, E. C. (2021, August 20). *Unemployment rates during the COVID-19 pandemic* (Report No. R46554). Congressional Research Service. Retrieved January 8, 2022, fromhttps://crsreports.congress.gov/product/details?prodcode=R46554

24. Why Did We Close Schools?

1. The coronavirus spring: The historic closing of U.S. schools (a timeline). (2020, July 1). *EducationWeek*. Retrieved January 8, 2022, from https://www.edweek.org/leadership/the-coronavirus-spring-the-historic-closing-of-u-s-schools-a-timeline/2020/07

2. Li, X., Xu, W., Dozier, M., He, Y., Kirolos, A., & Theodoratou, E. (2020). The role of children in transmission of SARS-CoV-2: A rapid review. *Journal of Global Health, 10*(1), 011101.

3. Rajmil, L. (2020). Role of children in the transmission of the COVID-19 pandemic: A rapid scoping review. *BMJ Paediatrics Open, 4*(1), e000722.

4. Götzinger, F., Santiago-García, B., Noguera-Julián, A., Lanaspa, M., Lancella, L., Calo Carducci, F., Gabrovska, N., Velizarova, S., Prunk, P., Osterman, V., Krivec, U., Lo Vecchio, A., Shingadia, D., Soriano-Arandes, A., Melendo, S., Lanari, M., Pierantoni, L., Wagner, N., L'Huillier, A., . . . Tebruegge, M.; ptbnet COVID-19 Study Group. (2020). COVID-19 in children and adolescents in Europe: A multinational, multicentre cohort study. *Lancet Child & Adolescent Health, 4*(9), 653–661.

5. Ludvigsson, J. F. (2020). Children are unlikely to be the main drivers of the COVID-19 pandemic—A systematic review. *Acta Paediatrica, 109*(8), 1525–1530.

6. Christakis, D. A., Van Cleve, W., & Zimmerman, F. J. (2020). Estimation of US children's educational attainment and years of life lost associated with primary school closures during the coronavirus disease 2019 pandemic. *JAMA Network Open, 3*(11), e202878.

7. Liesman, S. (2020, August 11). *Half of U.S. elementary and high school students will study virtually only this fall, study shows.* CNBC. Retrieved January 8, 2022, from https://www.cnbc.com/2020/08/11/half-of-us-elementary-and-high-school-students-will-study-virtually-only-this-fall-study-shows.html

8. U.S. Environmental Protection Agency. (n.d.). *How big a problem is poor indoor air quality (IAQ) in schools?* Retrieved January 8, 2022, fromhttps://www.epa.gov/iaq-schools/how-big-problem-poor-indoor-air-quality-iaq-schools

9. McDonald, K. (2020, November 9). Public school enrollment plummets as private schools see gains. *FEE Stories.* Retrieved January 8, 2022, from https://fee.org/articles/public-school-enrollment-plummets-as-private-schools-see-gains

25. The Limits of Our Tolerance

1. Centers for Disease Control and Prevention. (n.d.). *Stay up to date with your vaccines.* Retrieved January 8, 2022, from https://www.cdc.gov/coronavirus/2019-ncov/vaccines/stay-up-to-date.html?CDC_AA_refVal=https%3A%2F%2Fwww.cdc.gov%2Fcoronavirus%2F2019-ncov%2Fvaccines%2Ffully-vaccinated-guidance.html

2. Berry, C. R., Fowler, A., Glazer, T., Handel-Meyer, S., & MacMillen, A. (2021). Evaluating the effects of shelter-in-place policies during the COVID-19 pandemic. *Proceedings of the National Academy of Sciences of the USA, 118*(15), e202878.

26. Mismanaging Messages

1. Banco, E., Cancryn, A., Owermohle, S., & Gardner, L. (2021, September 24). *Booster confusion takes hold as Biden announces expanded eligibility.* Politico. Retrieved January 8, 2022, from https://www.politico.com/news/2021/09/24/biden-expanded-booster-rollout-514110

2. Steensels, D., Pierlet, N., Penders, J., Mesotten, D., & Heylen, L. (2021). Comparison of SARS-CoV-2 antibody response following vaccination with BNT162b2 and mRNA-1273. *JAMA, 326*(15), 1533–1535.

3. U.S. Food and Drug Administration. (2021, October 20). *Coronavirus (COVID-19) update: FDA takes additional actions on the use of a booster dose for COVID-19 vaccines.* Retrieved January 8, 2022, from https://www.fda. gov/news-events/press-announcements/coronavirus-COVID-19-upd ate-fda-takes-additional-actions-use-booster-dose-COVID-19-vaccines

4. Hamel, L., Lopes, L., Sparks, G., Kirzinger, A., Kearney, A., Stokes, M., & Brodie, M. (2021, September 28). *KFF COVID-19 vaccine monitor: September 2021.* KFF. Retrieved January 8, 2022, from https://www.kff.org/coronavi rus-COVID-19/poll-finding/kff-COVID-19-vaccine-monitor-septem ber-2021

27. The Vaccination Glass Half Full

1. Baicus, A. (2012). History of polio vaccination. *World Journal of Virology,* 1(4), 108–114.

2. Sirken, M. G. (1962). National participation trends, 1955–61, in the poliomyelitis vaccination program. *Public Health Reports, 77*(8), 661–670.

3. Lu, P.-J., Hung, M.-C., Srivastav, A., Grohskopf, L. A., Kobayashi, M., Harris, A. M., Dooling, K. L., Markowitz, L. E., Rodriquez-Lainz, A., & Williams, W. W. (2021, May 14). *Surveillance of vaccination coverage among adult populations—United States, 2018.* MMWR Morbidity and Mortality Weekly Report, 70(3), 1–26. Retrieved January 8, 2022, from https://www. cdc.gov/mmwr/volumes/70/ss/ss7003a1.htm

4. Heltzel, G., & Laurin, K. (2020). Polarization in America: Two possible futures. *Current Opinion in Behavioral Sciences, 34,* 179–184.

5. Span, P. (2022, October 22). Among seniors, a declining interest in boosters. *The New York Times.* Retrieved February 1, 2023, from https:// www.nytimes.com/2022/10/22/health/covid-vaccination-elde rly.html

Section 3. Ethics

28. Time for an Ethics Refresh?

1. Kramer, A. E. (2021, January 8). Why I got the Russian vaccine. *The New York Times.* Retrieved January 8, 2022, from https://www.nytimes. com/2021/01/08/world/europe/russian-vaccine.html

2. Reuters Staff. (2021, January 13). *Explainer: What's behind varying efficacy data for Sinovac's COVID-19 vaccine?* Reuters. Retrieved January 8, 2022, from

https://www.reuters.com/article/health-coronavirus-sinovac-explai
ner-int/explainer-whats-behind-varying-efficacy-data-for-sinovacs-
COVID-19-vaccine-idUSKBN29J0M1

3. Jones, I., & Roy P. (2021). Sputnik V COVID-19 vaccine candidate appears safe and effective. *Lancet, 397*(10275), 642–643.
4. Logunov, D. Y., Dolzhikova, I. V., Shcheblyakov, D. V., Tukhvatulin, A. I., Zubkova, O. V., & Dzharullaeva, A. S., Kovyrshina, A., Lubenets, N., Grousova, D., Erokhova, A., Botikov, A., Izhaeva, F., Popova, O., Ozharovskaya, T., Esmagambetov, I., Favorskaya, I., Zrelkin, D., Voronina, D., Shcherbinin, D., . . . Gintsburg, A.; Gam-COVID-Vac Vaccine Trial Group (2021). Safety and efficacy of an rAd26 and rAd5 vector-based heterologous prime-boost COVID-19 vaccine: An interim analysis of a randomised controlled phase 3 trial in Russia. *The Lancet, 397*(10275), 671–681.
5. Crimp, D. (2011, December 6). Before Occupy: How AIDS activists seized control of the FDA in 1988. *The Atlantic.* Retrieved January 8, 2022, from https://www.theatlantic.com/health/archive/2011/12/before-occupy-how-aids-activists-seized-control-of-the-fda-in-1988/249302
6. Doucleff, M. (2022, December 30). *China's COVID vaccines: Do the jabs do the job?* NPR. Retrieved February 1, 2023, from https://www.npr.org/sections/goatsandsoda/2022/12/30/1143696652/chinas-covid-vaccines-do-the-jabs-do-the-job

29. Who Goes First?

1. Markus, B. (2020, December 3). *The coronavirus vaccine is coming. That means planning for the largest vaccination effort in modern times.* CPR News. Retrieved January 8, 2022, from https://www.cpr.org/2020/12/03/we-know-coronavirus-vaccines-are-getting-close-we-arent-sure-who-will-get-them-first
2. Hutchinson, A., & José, R. R. (2020, December 15). *ADH COVID-19 vaccination phased plan.* Arkansas Department of Health. Retrieved January 8, 2022, fromhttps://www.healthy.arkansas.gov/images/uploads/pdf/HAN-covid_phased_plan_12_15Final.pdf
3. Georgia Department of Public Health. (n.d.). *COVID-19 vaccines: Safe. Tested. Effective.* Retrieved January 8, 2022, from https://dph.georgia.gov/covid-vaccine

30. What's Most Important?

1. Johnson & Johnson. (27, February 2021). *Johnson & Johnson COVID-19 vaccine authorized by U.S. FDA for emergency use—First single-shot vaccine in fight against global pandemic.* Retrieved January 8, 2022, from https://www.jnj.com/johnson-johnson-COVID-19-vaccine-authorized-by-u-s-fda-for-emergency-usefirst-single-shot-vaccine-in-fight-against-global-pandemic

31. Achieving Health Equity, Efficiently

1. Stein, M. D., & Galea, S. (2020). *Pained: Uncomfortable conversations about the public's health.* Oxford University Press.
2. National Academies of Science, Engineering, and Medicine. (n.d.). *A framework for equitable allocation of vaccine for the novel coronavirus.* Retrieved January 8, 2022, from https://www.nationalacademies.org/our-work/a-framework-for-equitable-allocation-of-vaccine-for-the-novel-coronavirus
3. Centers for Disease Control and Prevention. (2020, December 3). *COVID-19 ACIP vaccine recommendations.* Retrieved January 10, 2022, from https://www.cdc.gov/vaccines/hcp/acip-recs/vacc-specific/COVID-19.html
4. *Coronavirus NY: State will fine $1M for coronavirus vaccine fraud.* (2020, December 28). ABC 7 NY. Retrieved January 10, 2022, from https://abc7ny.com/parcare-vaccine-fraud-attorney-general-ny-covid/9143911
5. New York's COVID vaccine sites are open—but largely empty—after midnight. (2021, January 14). *The Wall Street Journal.* Retrieved January 10, 2022, from https://www.wsj.com/story/new-york-covid-vaccine-sites-are-openbut-largely-emptyafter-midnight-d5e86dbe
6. Stern, J. (2021, January 13). Random people are lining up to get vaccinated in D.C. grocery stores. *The Atlantic.* Retrieved January 10, 2022, from https://www.theatlantic.com/health/archive/2021/01/COVID-19-vaccine-giveaways-are-getting-out-control/617669
7. Rubinstein, D. (2021, January 10). After unused vaccines are thrown in trash, Cuomo loosens rules. *The New York Times.* Retrieved January 10, 2022, from https://www.nytimes.com/2021/01/10/nyregion/new-york-vaccine-guidelines.html

33. Health Inequities Beyond COVID-19

1. Woolf, S. H., Chapman, D. A., & Lee, J. H. (2021). COVID-19 as the leading cause of death in the United States. *JAMA, 325*(2), 123–124.
2. *Number of deaths involving coronavirus disease 2019 (COVID-19), pneumonia, and influenza in the U.S.* (n.d.). Statista. Retrieved January 10, 2022, from https://www.statista.com/statistics/1113051/number-reported-deaths-from-covid-pneumonia-and-flu-us
3. Centers for Disease Control and Prevention. (n.d.). *FastStats—Death and mortality.* Retrieved January 10, 2022, from https://www.cdc.gov/nchs/fastats/deaths.htm
4. The COVID Tracking Project. (n.d.). *The COVID racial data tracker.* Retrieved January 10, 2022, from https://covidtracking.com/race
5. Centers for Disease Control and Prevention. (n.d.). *Health equity considerations and racial and ethnic minority groups.* Retrieved January 10, 2022, from https://www.cdc.gov/coronavirus/2019-ncov/community/health-equity/race-ethnicity.html
6. Egede, L. E., & Walker, R. J. (2020). Structural racism, social risk factors, and COVID-19—A dangerous convergence for Black Americans. *New England Journal of Medicine, 383,* e77.
7. Maani, N., & Galea, S. (2020). COVID-19 and underinvestment in the health of the US population. *Milbank Quarterly, 98*(2), 239–249.
8. Wrigley-Field, E. (2020). US racial inequality may be as deadly as COVID-19. *Proceedings of the National Academy of Sciences of the USA, 117*(36), 21854–21856.

34. A Hard Weight

1. World Obesity. (2021, March). *COVID-19 and obesity: The 2021 atlas.* Retrieved January 10, 2022, from https://www.worldobesityday.org/assets/downloads/COVID-19-and-Obesity-The-2021-Atlas.pdf
2. Department of Health & Social Care. (2020, July 27). *Tackling obesity: Empowering adults and children to live healthier lives.* GOV.UK. Retrieved January 10, 2022, from https://www.gov.uk/government/publications/tackling-obesity-government-strategy/tackling-obesity-empowering-adults-and-children-to-live-healthier-lives

35. Mandating Vaccines

1. Dolgin, E. (2021). The tangled history of mRNA vaccines. *Nature*, *597*(7876), 318–324.
2. Miller, Z. (2021, June 15). *"A summer of freedom": Vaccine gives new meaning to July 4th*. The Associated Press. Retrieved January 10, 2022, from https://apnews.com/article/government-and-politics-joe-biden-lifestyle-coronavirus-pandemic-health-f97e0316c51d2d8362a17d149daedb14
3. John, P. R., Heith, K., Johnson, E. M., & Gaeta, M. S. (2021, June 17). *Ethical considerations for a COVID-19 vaccine mandate*. Society of Critical Care and Medicine. Retrieved January 10, 2022, from https://www.sccm.org/Blog/June-2021/Ethical-Considerations-for-a-COVID-19-Vaccine-Mand

36. Leaving the World Behind

1. USAFacts. (n.d.). *US coronavirus vaccine tracker*. Retrieved January 10, 2022, from https://usafacts.org/visualizations/covid-vaccine-tracker-states
2. Coronavirus (COVID-19) vaccinations. (n.d.). *Our World in Data*. Retrieved January 10, 2022, from https://ourworldindata.org/covid-vaccinations
3. Roser, M., Ortiz-Ospina, E., & Ritchie, H. (2019, October). Life expectancy. *Our World in Data*. Retrieved January 10, 2022, from https://ourworldindata.org/life-expectancy
4. Abdalla, S. M., Allotey, P., Ettman, C. K., Galea, S., Maani, N., Parsey, L., & Rhule, E. (2021, September). *Task Force 1: Global health and COVID-19—Global equity for global health*. Think20 Italy. Retrieved January 10, 2022, from https://www.t20italy.org/2021/09/08/global-equity-for-global-health
5. Keaten, J. (2021, September 8). *WHO chief urges halt to booster shots for rest of the year*. The Associated Press. Retrieved January 10, 2022, from https://apnews.com/article/business-health-coronavirus-pandemic-united-nations-world-health-organization-6384ff91c399679824311ac26e3c768a

37. Digital Surveillance

1. *Publicly-available exposure notifications apps*. (n.d.). Google API for Exposure Notifications. Retrieved January 10, 2022, from https://developers.google.com/android/exposure-notifications/apps

2. Dayaram, S. (2020, March 22). *Singapore's coronavirus playbook: How it fought back against the COVID-19 pandemic.* CNET. Retrieved January 10, 2022, from https://www.cnet.com/health/singapores-coronavirus-playbook-how-one-country-fought-back-against-covid19-epidemic

3. McCurry, J. (2020, April 22). Test, trace, contain: How South Korea flattened its coronavirus curve. *The Guardian.* Retrieved January 10, 2022, from https://www.theguardian.com/world/2020/apr/23/test-trace-cont ain-how-south-korea-flattened-its-coronavirus-curve

4. *Israel: Security service may use patients' smartphone data for contact tracing.* (2020, March 17). Privacy International. Retrieved January 10, 2022, from https://privacyinternational.org/examples/3423/israel-security-service-may-use-patients-smartphone-data-contact-tracing

5. Valade, P. (2020, May 21). *Jumbo Privacy review: North Dakota's contact tracing app.* Jumbo Privacy. Retrieved January 10, 2022, from https://blog.jumbo privacy.com/jumbo-privacy-review-north-dakota-s-contact-tracing-app.html

6. American Civil Liberties Union. (2021, July 15). *The fight to stop face recognition technology.* Retrieved January 10, 2022, from https://www.aclu.org/news/topic/stopping-face-recognition-surveillance

7. Whittaker, Z. (2020, August 19). *Fearing coronavirus, a Michigan college is tracking its students with a flawed app.* Tech Crunch. Retrieved January 10, 2022, from https://techcrunch.com/2020/08/19/coronavirus-albion-security-flaws-app

8. Jewell, C. (2019, June). *Artificial intelligence: The new electricity.* World Intellectual Property Organization. Retrieved January 10, 2022, from https://www.wipo.int/wipo_magazine/en/2019/03/article_0001.html

38. Balancing Autonomy and Individual Responsibility

1. Fairchild, A. L., Healton, C., & Galea, S. (2020, July 15). *A national mandatory order to wear a mask would keep people from becoming "walking weapons."* STAT. Retrieved January 10, 2022, from https://www.statnews.com/2020/07/15/national-mandatory-mask-order-prevent-walking-weapons

2. Centers for Disease Control and Prevention. (n.d.). *Guidance for wearing masks.* Retrieved January 10, 2022, from https://www.cdc.gov/coronavi rus/2019-ncov/prevent-getting-sick/cloth-face-cover-guidance.html

3. Centers for Disease Control and Prevention. (n.d.). *Smokefree policies reduce secondhand smoke exposure.* Retrieved January 10, 2022, from https://www.cdc.gov/tobacco/data_statistics/fact_sheets/secondhand_smoke/protection/shs_exposure/index.htm

4. Markowitz, A. (n.d.). *State-by-state guide to face mask requirements.* AARP. Retrieved January 10, 2022, from https://www.aarp.org/health/healthy-living/info-2020/states-mask-mandates-coronavirus.html

5. Fairchild, A. L., Healton, C., Galea, S., Holtgrave, D., & Curran, J. W. (2021, March 9). To end the pandemic faster, don't give up on state mask policies. *Governing.* Retrieved January 10, 2022, from https://www.governing.com/now/to-end-the-pandemic-faster-dont-give-up-on-state-mask-policies.html

6. Institute of Medicine. (2002). *The future of the public's health in the 21st century.* National Academies Press.

39. Profits and Profiteering

1. Togini, G. (2021, April 6). Meet the 40 new billionaires who got rich fighting COVID-19. *Forbes.* Retrieved January 10, 2022, from https://www.forbes.com/sites/giacomotognini/2021/04/06/meet-the-40-new-billionaires-who-got-rich-fighting-COVID-19/?sh=26ed7a7e17e5

2. Satija, N., & Sun, L. H. (2019, December 20). A major funder of the anti-vaccine movement has made millions selling natural health products. *The Washington Post.* Retrieved January 10, 2022, from https://www.washingtonpost.com/investigations/2019/10/15/fdc01078-c29c-11e9-b5e4-54aa56d5b7ce_story.html

3. U.S. Food & Drug Administration. (n.d.). *Why you should not use ivermectin to treat or prevent COVID-19.* Retrieved January 10, 2022, from https://www.fda.gov/consumers/consumer-updates/why-you-should-not-use-ivermectin-treat-or-prevent-COVID-19#:~:text=You%20can%20also%20overdose%20on,seizures%2C%20coma%20and%20even%20death

4. Hennekens, C. H., Rane, M., Solano, J., Alter, S., Johnson, H., Krishnaswamy, S., Shih, R., Maki, D., & DeMets, D. (2021). Updates on hydroxychloroquine in prevention and treatment of COVID-19. *American Journal of Medicine, 135*(1), 7–9.

5. Dilanian, K., Ramgopal, K., & Atkins, C. (2021, August 15). "Easy money": How international scam artists pulled off an epic theft of Covid benefits. NBC News. Retrieved January 10, 2022, from https://www.nbcnews.com/news/us-news/easy-money-how-international-scam-artists-pulled-epic-theft-covid-n1276789

6. Robbins, R. (2021, October 9). Moderna, racing for profits, keeps Covid vaccine out of reach of poor. *The New York Times.* Retrieved January 10, 2022, from https://www.nytimes.com/2021/10/09/business/moderna-covid-vaccine.html?campaign_id=9&campaign_id=154&emc=

edit_cb_20211011&instance_id=42511&instance_id=42581&nl=coro
navirus-briefing&regi_id=93388816&regi_id=79204246&segment_id=
71276&segment_id=71354&te=1&

Section 4. Emotions

41. Recognizing and Moving Beyond Our Collective Grief

1. United States COVID–Coronavirus statistics. (n.d.). Worldometer.
   Retrieved January 10, 2022, from https://www.worldometers.info/coro
   navirus/country/us
2. Gonzalez, O. (2021, February 23). *Axios–Ipsos poll: 1 in 3 Americans know*
   someone who died from COVID-19. Axios. Retrieved January 10, 2022, from
   https://www.axios.com/coronavirus-death-know-someone-263d12d2-
   9296-4547-8d57-e619f65d47e2.html
3. Keyes, K. M., Pratt, C., Galea, S., McLaughlin, K. A., Koenen, K. C., &
   Shear, M. K. (2014). The burden of loss: Unexpected death of a loved
   one and psychiatric disorders across the life course in a national study.
   American Journal of Psychiatry, 171(8), 864–871.
4. Panchal, N., Kamal, R., Cox, C., & Garfield, R. (2021, February 10). *The*
   implications of COVID-19 for mental health and substance use. KFF. Retrieved
   January 10, 2022, from https://www.kff.org/coronavirus-COVID-19/
   issue-brief/the-implications-of-COVID-19-for-mental-health-and-
   substance-use
5. Ettman, C. K., Abdalla, S. M., Cohen, G. H., Sampson, L., Vivier, P. M., &
   Galea, S. (2020). Prevalence of depression symptoms in US adults before
   and during the COVID-19 pandemic. *JAMA, 3*(9), e2019686.
6. National September 11 Memorial & Museum. (n.d.). *9/11 Memorial &*
   Museum. Retrieved January 10, 2022, from https://www.911memorial.
   org/learn

42. Epistemic Humility During a Global Pandemic

1. Joseph, A. (2021, March 17). *Driven by the pandemic and "the Fauci effect,"*
   applicants flood public health schools. STAT. Retrieved January 10, 2022, from
   https://www.statnews.com/2021/03/17/driven-by-pandemic-applica
   nts-flood-public-health-schools
2. Senior, J. (2020, March 9). *President Trump is unfit for this crisis. Period. The*
   New York Times. Retrieved January 10, 2022, from https://www.nytimes.
   com/2020/03/09/opinion/trump-corona-cdc.html

3. Miller, C. C., Sanger-Katz, M., & Bui, Q. (2020, November 20). *What 635 epidemiologists are doing for Thanksgiving. The New York Times.* Retrieved January 10, 2022, from https://www.nytimes.com/2020/11/20/upshot/how-epidemiologists-spending-thanksgiving.html

4. Bock, M. (n.d.). *A surge in public health related careers would be a welcome response to this pandemic.* CollegiateParent. Retrieved January 10, 2022, from https://www.collegiateparent.com/career/public-health-careers-response-to-the-pandemic

5. *Model used to evaluate lockdowns was flawed.* (2020, December 26). Lund University. Retrieved January 10, 2022, from https://www.lunduniversity.lu.se/article/model-used-evaluate-lockdowns-was-flawed

6. Pike, L. (2020, May 9). Why 15 US states suddenly made masks mandatory. *Vox.* Retrieved January 10, 2022, from https://www.vox.com/2020/5/29/21273625/coronavirus-masks-required-virginia-china-hong-kong

7. Jackson, D. Z. (2020, October 23). *Herding people to slaughter: The dangerous fringe theory behind the Great Barrington Declaration and push toward herd immunity.* Union of Concerned Scientists. Retrieved January 10, 2022, from https://blog.ucsusa.org/derrick-jackson/herding-people-to-slaughter-the-dangerous-fringe-theory-behind-the-great-barrington-declaration-and-push-toward-herd-immunity

8. *Great Barrington Declaration.* (2020). Retrieved January 10, 2022, from https://gbdeclaration.org

43. The Selling of Vaccines

1. Centers for Disease Control and Prevention. (n.d.). *COVID-19 vaccinations in the United States.* Retrieved January 10, 2022, from https://covid.cdc.gov/covid-data-tracker/#vaccinations_vacc-total-admin-rate-total

2. Coronavirus (COVID-19) vaccinations. (n.d.). *Our World in Data.* Retrieved January 10, 2022, from https://ourworldindata.org/covid-vaccinations

3. Ompad, D. C., Galea, S., & Vlahov, D. (2006). Distribution of influenza vaccine to high-risk groups. *Epidemiologic Reviews, 28,* 54–70.

45. Hope Dies Last

1. Camus, A. (1991). *The plague* (S. Gilbert, Trans.). Vintage. (Original translation published 1948)

2. Shapiro, A. (2020, April 8). "*The Plague*" is a top seller as fiction sales drop during coronavirus shutdowns. *Forbes.* Retrieved January 10, 2022, from

https://www.forbes.com/sites/arielshapiro/2020/04/08/the-plague-is-a-top-seller-as-fiction-sales-drop-during-coronavirus-shutdowns/?sh=42511086aa55

3. James, L. P., Salomon, J. A., Buckee, C. O., & Menzies, N. A. (2021). The use and misuse of mathematical modeling for infectious disease policymaking: Lessons for the COVID-19 pandemic. *Medical Decision Making*, 41(4), 379–385.

4. Wallace-Wells, B. (2021, August 12). What happened to Joe Biden's "summer of freedom" from the pandemic? *The New Yorker*. Retrieved January 10, 2022, from https://www.newyorker.com/news/annals-of-inquiry/what-happened-to-joe-bidens-summer-of-freedom-from-the-pandemic

5. Casselman, B. (2020, July 30). *A collapse that wiped out 5 years of growth, with no bounce in sight. The New York Times*. Retrieved January 10, 2022, from https://www.nytimes.com/2020/07/30/business/economy/q2-gdp-coronavirus-economy.html

6. Nearly one-fifth of Americans know someone who has died of COVID-19, survey says. (2021, March 11). *uchicago news*. Retrieved January 10, 2022, from https://news.uchicago.edu/story/nearly-one-fifth-americans-know-someone-who-has-died-COVID-19-survey-says

46. Can We Forget?

1. Woolf, S. H., Chapman, D. A., Sabo, R. T., Weinberger, D. M., Hill, L., & Taylor, D. D. (2020). Excess deaths from COVID-19 and other causes, March–July 2020. *JAMA*, 324(15), 1562–1564.

2. Roberts, L. (2021). How COVID hurt the fight against other dangerous diseases. *Nature*, 592(7855), 502–504.

3. Adamy, J. (2021, December 22). Life expectancy in U.S. declined 1.8 years in 2020, CDC says. *The Wall Street Journal*. Retrieved January 11, 2022, from https://www.wsj.com/articles/life-expectancy-in-u-s-declined-1-8-years-in-2020-cdc-says-11640149261

4. Falk, G., Romero, P. D., Nicchitta, I. A., & Nyhof, E. C. (2021, August 20). *Unemployment rates during the COVID-19 pandemic* (Report No. R46554). Congressional Research Service. Retrieved January 11, 2022, from https://crsreports.congress.gov/product/details?prodcode=R46554

5. Whitman, W. (n.d.). *Published works: Books by Whitman*. The Walt Whitman Archive. Retrieved January 11, 2022, from https://whitmanarchive.org/published/LG/1891/poems/41

47. The Centrality of Compassion

1. Galea, S. (2018). The complicity of the population health scientist. *Milbank Quarterly*, 96(2), 227–230.

50. Trust and COVID-19

1. Arrow, K. J. (1974). *The limits of organization*. Norton.
2. Rainie, L., & Perrin, A. (2019, July 22). *Key findings about Americans' declining trust in government and each other*. Pew Research Center. Retrieved January 11, 2022, from https://www.pewresearch.org/fact-tank/2019/07/22/key-findings-about-americans-declining-trust-in-government-and-each-other
3. Simmons-Duffin, S. (2021, May 13). *Poll finds public health has a trust problem*. NPR. Retrieved January 11, 2022, from https://www.npr.org/2021/05/13/996331692/poll-finds-public-health-has-a-trust-problem
4. Baker, M., & Ivory, D. (2021, October 18). Why public health faces a crisis across the U.S. *The New York Times*. Retrieved January 11, 2022, from https://www.nytimes.com/2021/10/18/us/coronavirus-public-health.html

Section 5. The Future

51. The New Us?

1. Rogers, K. (2010, February 25). *1968 flu pandemic*. Britannica. Retrieved January 11, 2022, from https://www.britannica.com/event/1968-flu-pandemic
2. Spinney, L. (2020, March 7). The world changed its approach to health after the 1918 flu. Will it after the COVID-19 outbreak? *TIME*. Retrieved January 11, 2022, from https://time.com/5797629/health-1918-flu-epidemic

52. Who Decides?

1. Insurance Institute for Highway Safety and Highway Loss Data Institute. (2019, April 4). *Speed limit increases are tied to 37,000 deaths over 25 years*. Retrieved January 11, 2022, from https://www.iihs.org/news/detail/speed-limit-increases-are-tied-to-37-000-deaths-over-25-years

2. Government of Canada. (2019). *Canadian motor vehicle traffic collision statistics: 2018.* Retrieved January 11, 2022, from https://tc.canada.ca/en/road-transportation/statistics-data/canadian-motor-vehicle-traffic-collision-statistics-2018

3. Insurance Institute for Highway Safety and Highway Loss Data Institute. (2021, March). *Fatality facts 2019 state by state.* Retrieved January 11, 2022, from https://www.iihs.org/topics/fatality-statistics/detail/state-by-state

4. Galea, S., & Vaughan, R. (2021). Embedding prevention at the heart of the US health conversation. *American Journal of Public Health, 111*(1), 17–19.

54. HIV and COVID-19

1. Kramer, L. (2020, May 27). *1,112 and counting.* Longform. Retrieved January 11, 2022, from https://longform.org/posts/1-112-and-counting

2. Walker, N. (2020, July 1). Drug approval trends: Significant acceleration in recent years. *Pharma's Almanac.* Retrieved January 11, 2022, from https://www.pharmasalmanac.com/articles/drug-approval-trends-significant-acceleration-in-recent-years

3. Lippman, D., & McGraw, M. (2020, April 2). *Inside the National Security Council, a rising sense of dread.* Politico. Retrieved January 11, 2022, from https://www.politico.com/news/2020/04/02/nsc-coronavirus-white-house-162530

4. Spencer, J., Guardian, T., & Jewett, C. (2021, April 8). *12 months of trauma: More than 3,600 US health workers died in Covid's first year.* KHN. Retrieved January 11, 2022, from https://khn.org/news/article/us-health-workers-deaths-covid-lost-on-the-frontline/#:~:text=our%20Privacy%20Policy

55. Guns and the Unanticipated Consequences of COVID-19

1. Gun Violence Archive. (2021). *Gun violence archive.* Retrieved January 7, 2022, from https://www.gunviolencearchive.org

2. Uvalde school shooting. (2022). *The Texas Tribune.* Retrieved August 10, 2022, from https://www.texastribune.org/series/uvalde-texas-school-shooting

56. Policies That Persist

1. Castrodale, J. (2021, June 17). U.S. alcohol sales in 2020 were at their highest levels in 18 years. *Food & Wine*. Retrieved January 11, 2022, from https://www.foodandwine.com/news/usa-alcohol-sales-in-2020
2. Pollard, M. S., Tucker, J. S., & Green, H. D. (2020). Changes in adult alcohol use and consequences during the COVID-19 pandemic in the US. *JAMA Network Open, 3*(9), e2022942.
3. Kushner, T. (2020). Chronic liver disease and COVID-19: Alcohol use disorder/alcohol-associated liver disease, nonalcoholic fatty liver disease/nonalcoholic steatohepatitis, autoimmune liver disease, and compensated cirrhosis. *Clinical Liver Disease, 15*(5), 195–199.
4. Chalfin, A., Danagoulian, S., & Deza, M. (2021, March). *COVID-19 has strengthened the relationship between alcohol consumption and domestic violence.* National Bureau of Economic Research. Retrieved January 11, 2022, from https://www.nber.org/papers/w28523

57. The Invisible Work of Public Health

1. *Fact sheet: Biden–Harris administration to invest $7 billion from American Rescue Plan to hire and train public health workers in response to COVID- 19.* (2021, May 13). The White House. Retrieved January 11, 2022, from https://www.whitehouse.gov/briefing-room/statements-releases/2021/05/13/fact-sheet-biden-harris-administration-to-invest-7-billion-from-american-rescue-plan-to-hire-and-train-public-health-workers-in-response-to-COVID-19
2. Begley, S. (2020, April 2). *COVID-19 spreads too fast for traditional contact tracing. New digital tools could help.* STAT. Retrieved January 11, 2022, from https://www.statnews.com/2020/04/02/coronavirus-spreads-too-fast-for-contact-tracing-digital-tools-could-help
3. Maani, N., & Galea, S. (2020). COVID-19 and underinvestment in the public health infrastructure of the United States. *Milbank Quarterly, 98*(2), 250–259.
4. Torton, B. (2021, January 25). *Legal protections for public health officials during the COVID-19 pandemic.* The Network for Public Health Law. Retrieved January 11, 2022, from https://www.networkforphl.org/resources/legal-protections-for-public-health-officials-during-COVID-19

5. Simmons-Duffin, S. (2021, May 13). *Poll finds public health has a trust problem.* NPR. Retrieved January 11, 2022, from https://www.npr.org/2021/05/13/996331692/poll-finds-public-health-has-a-trust-problem

58. Will Better Public Health Funding Be Enough?

1. Maani, N., & Galea, S. (2020). COVID-19 and underinvestment in the public health infrastructure of the United States. *Milbank Quarterly, 98*(2), 250–259.
2. Weber, L., Ungar, L., Smith, M. R., Recht, H., Barry-Jester, A. M., & The Associated Press. (2020, July 1). *Hollowed-out public health system faces more cuts amid virus.* KHN. Retrieved January 11, 2022, from https://khn.org/news/us-public-health-system-underfunded-under-threat-faces-more-cuts-amid-covid-pandemic
3. Association of Schools of Public Health. (2008, December). *ASPH policy brief: Confronting the public health workforce crisis.* Retrieved January 11, 2022, from https://www.healthpolicyfellows.org/pdfs/ConfrontingthePublicHealthWorkforceCrisisbyASPH.pdf
4. Wilson, R. T., Troisi, C. L., & Gary-Webb, T. L. (2020, April 5). *A deficit of more than 250,000 public health workers is no way to fight COVID-19.* STAT. Retrieved January 11, 2022, from https://www.statnews.com/2020/04/05/deficit-public-health-workers-no-way-to-fight-COVID-19
5. *Fact Sheet: Biden–Harris administration to invest $7 billion from American Rescue Plan to hire and train public health workers in response to COVID- 19.* (2021, May 13). The White House. Retrieved January 11, 2022, from https://www.whitehouse.gov/briefing-room/statements-releases/2021/05/13/fact-sheet-biden-harris-administration-to-invest-7-billion-from-american-rescue-plan-to-hire-and-train-public-health-workers-in-response-to-COVID-19
6. Beitsch, L. M., Castrucci, B. C., Dilley, A., Leider, J., Juliano, C., Nelson, R., Kaiman, S., & Sprague, J. (2014). From patchwork to package: Implementing foundational capabilities for state and local health departments. *American Journal of Public Health, 105*(2), e7–e10.
7. Stein, M., & Galea, S. (2021, June 24). *Health inequities beyond COVID-19.* Public Health Post. Retrieved January 11, 2022, from https://www.publichealthpost.org/the-turning-point/health-inequities-beyond-COVID-19

8. DeSalvo, K., Hughes, B., Bassett, M., Benjamin, G., Fraser, M., Galea, S., & Gracia, J. N. (2021). Public health COVID-19 impact assessment: Lessons learned and compelling needs. *NAM Perspectives, 2021*, 10.31478/202104c.

59. Chronic COVID

1. Lam, M. H.-B., Wing, Y.-K., Yu, M. W.-M., Leung, C. M., Ma, R. C., Kong, A. P., So, W. Y., Fong, S. Y., & Lam, S. P. (2009). Mental morbidities and chronic fatigue in severe acute respiratory syndrome survivors: Long-term follow-up. *Archives of Internal Medicine, 169*(22), 2142–2147.
2. Gaffney, A. W. (2021, March 22). *We need to start thinking more critically—and speaking more cautiously—about long Covid.* STAT. Retrieved January 11, 2022, from https://www.statnews.com/2021/03/22/we-need-to-start-thinking-more-critically-speaking-cautiously-long-covid
3. Centers for Disease Control and Prevention. (n.d.). *Nearly one in five American adults who have had COVID-19 still have "long COVID."* Retrieved February 1, 2023, from https://www.cdc.gov/nchs/pressroom/nchs_pre ss_releases/2022/20220622.htm
4. Centers for Disease Control and Prevention. (n.d.). *Long COVID or post-COVID conditions.* Centers for Disease Control and Prevention. Retrieved February 1, 2023, from https://www.cdc.gov/coronavirus/2019-ncov/long-term-effects/index.html
5. Belluck, P. (2022, June 25). *New research hints at 4 factors that may increase chances of long Covid.* The New York Times. Retrieved February 1, 2023, from https://www.nytimes.com/2022/01/25/health/long-covid-risk-fact ors.html

60. COVID-19 Collectivism

1. Survivor Corps.(n.d.). [Home page]. Retrieved January 11, 2022, from https://www.survivorcorps.com
2. Long COVID Alliance. (n.d.). [Home page]. Retrieved January 11, 2022, fromhttps://longcovidalliance.org

61. Can We Be Led?

1. Biden, J. R. (2021, February 24). *Notice on the continuation of the national emergency concerning the coronavirus disease 2019 (COVID- 19) pandemic.* The

White House. Retrieved January 11, 2022, from https://www.whiteho
use.gov/briefing-room/presidential-actions/2021/02/24/notice-on-the-
continuation-of-the-national-emergency-concerning-the-coronavirus-
disease-2019-COVID-19-pandemic

2. Wallace-Wells, B. (2021, August 12). *What happened to Joe Biden's "summer of freedom" from the pandemic? The New Yorker.* Retrieved January 11, 2022, from https://www.newyorker.com/news/annals-of-inquiry/what-happened-to-joe-bidens-summer-of-freedom-from-the-pandemic

3. Howard, J. (2021, November 8). *What the end of the COVID-19 pandemic could look like.* CNN. Retrieved January 11, 2022, from https://www.cnn.com/2021/11/08/health/COVID-19-pandemic-endgame-wellness/index.html

4. Centers for Disease Control and Prevention. (n.d.). *COVID-19 risks and vaccine information for older adults.*. Retrieved January 11, 2022, from https://www.cdc.gov/aging/covid19/covid19-older-adults.html

62. COVID-19 and the Office

1. Gould, E., & Shierholz, H. (2020, March 19). *Not everybody can work from home.* Economic Policy Institute. Retrieved January 11, 2022, from https://www.epi.org/blog/black-and-hispanic-workers-are-much-less-likely-to-be-able-to-work-from-home

2. *History of the organization of work: The craft guilds.* (n.d.). Britannica. Retrieved January 11, 2022, from https://www.britannica.com/topic/history-of-work-organization-648000/The-craft-guilds

3. A shield for employers: State COVID-19 indemnity laws: November 2020. (2020, November 30). *The National Law Review.* Retrieved January 11, 2022, from https://www.natlawreview.com/article/shield-employers-state-COVID-19-indemnity-laws-november-2020

4. Centers for Disease Control and Prevention. (n.d.). *COVID-19 employer information for office buildings.* Retrieved January 11, 2022, from https://www.cdc.gov/coronavirus/2019-ncov/community/office-buildings.html

5. U.S. Bureau of Labor Statistics. (n.d.). *Labor force statistics from the Current Population Survey.* Retrieved January 11, 2022, from https://www.bls.gov/cps/effects-of-the-coronavirus-COVID-19-pandemic.htm#MayJune

6. U.S. Bureau of Labor Statistics. (2021, August). *Economic news release.* Retrieved January 11, 2022, from https://www.bls.gov/news.release/archives/empsit_09032021.htm

63. A COVID-19 Poverty Surprise

1. Fox, L., & Burns, K. (2021, September 14). *The Supplemental Poverty Measure: 2020.* U.S. Census Bureau. Retrieved January 11, 2022, from https://www.census.gov/library/publications/2021/demo/p60-275.html
2. Confronting Poverty. (n.d.). *Poverty facts and myths.* Retrieved January 11, 2022, from https://confrontingpoverty.org/poverty-facts-and-myths/most-americans-will-experience-poverty
3. Graham, C. (2020, November 17). *The human costs of the pandemic: Is it time to prioritize well-being?* Brookings. Retrieved January 11, 2022, from https://www.brookings.edu/research/the-human-costs-of-the-pandemic-is-it-time-to-prioritize-well-being
4. Long, H., & Goldstein, A. (2021, September 14). Poverty fell overall in 2020 as result of massive stimulus checks and unemployment aid, Census Bureau says. *The Washington Post.* Retrieved January 11, 2022, from https://www.washingtonpost.com/business/2021/09/14/us-census-poverty-health-insurance-2020
5. Coleman-Jensen, A., Rabbitt, M. P., Gregory, C. A., & Singh, A. (2021, September). *Household food security in the United States in 2020.* U.S. Department of Agriculture, Economic Research Service. Retrieved January 11, 2022, from https://www.ers.usda.gov/webdocs/publications/102076/err-298.pdf?v=5663.5
6. The National Academies of Sciences, Engineering, and Medicine. (2019). *A roadmap to reducing child poverty.* National Academies Press.

64. Is It Over Yet?

1. Centers for Disease Control and Prevention. (2020, October 1). *Past seasons estimated influenza disease burden.* Retrieved January 11, 2022, from https://www.cdc.gov/flu/about/burden/past-seasons.html
2. Weixel, N. (2020, June 15). Trump on coronavirus: "If we stop testing right now, we'd have very few cases, if any." *The Hill.* Retrieved January 11, 2022, from https://thehill.com/policy/healthcare/502819-trump-on-coronavirus-if-we-stop-testing-right-now-wed-have-very-few-cases
3. Hamer, D. H., White, L. F., Jenkins, H. E., Gill, C. J., Landsberg, H. E., Klapperich, C., Bulekova, K., Platt, J., Decarie, L., Gilmore, W., Pilkington, M., MacDowell, T. L., Faria, M. A., Densmore, D., Landaverde, L., Li, W., Rose, T., Burgay, S. P., Miller, C., . . . Brown, R. A. (2021). Assessment of a COVID-19 control plan on an urban university campus during a second wave of the pandemic. *JAMA Network Open, 4*(6), e2116425.

4. Kamp, J. (2020, September 19). *Death toll from COVID-19 pandemic extends far beyond virus victims. The Wall Street Journal.* Retrieved January 11, 2022, from https://www.wsj.com/articles/death-toll-from-COVID-19-pandemic-extends-far-beyond-virus-victims-11600507800

65. Now What?

1. Total confirmed COVID-19 cases. (n.d.). *Our World in Data.* Retrieved January 11, 2022, from https://ourworldindata.org/search?q=total+covid+cases
2. Chen, J., & McGeorge, R. (2020, October 23). Spillover effects of the COVID-19 pandemic could drive long-term health consequences for non-COVID-19 patients. *Health Affairs.* Retrieved January 11, 2022, from https://www.healthaffairs.org/do/10.1377/forefront.20201020.566558/full
3. Coronavirus (COVID-19) vaccinations. (n.d.). *Our World in Data.* Retrieved January 11, 2022, from https://ourworldindata.org/covid-vaccinations
4. Centers for Disease Control and Prevention. (n.d.). *COVID data tracker.* Retrieved February 1, 2023, from https://covid.cdc.gov/covid-data-tracker/#datatracker-home
5. World Health Organization. (n.d.). *WHO coronavirus (COVID-19) dashboard.* Retrieved February 1, 2023, from https://covid19.who.int